"Brent's Christian faith has led him to make this profound, warmly readable book about psychoanalysis and its future. His study of faith, including a remarkably healing case study, takes us away from fallacious assumptions that suffering should be pathologized and salvation must be found merely through human cleverness and social engineering."

John Gordon, *Author of* Healing Madness

"This book comes alive with faith in many dimensions. It breathes, aches, suffers, cries and opens depths of joy and renewal. It speaks of a wound that lights and gives credit to much that is devalued, including creative aspects of madness and such pages that keep giving."

Michael Eigen, PhD., *Author of books including* The Challenge of Being Human, The Psychotic Core, Contact with the Depths, Faith, and The Psychoanalytic Mystic

"In the face of fracture and contentious uncertainty we are easily seduced by certitude, tempted to abandon our doubt in the chimeric fortress of knowledge. But at what cost? In his new book Elements of Faith, Brent Potter takes us into the psychoanalytic situation, not as a contender to faith, but as a handmaid in the service of fostering our capacities to embrace mystery, meaning, and courageous openness. Of course we need knowledge, but Potter's invitation is to walk into the vitalizing tensions of knowing and not knowing, the already and the not yet, the world we inhabit and the world yet to be."

Earl D. Bland, PsyD, Psy, *Professor of Psychology, Licensed Psychologist/Psychoanalyst, Rosemead School of Psychology*

"In a time when we are seeing a resurgence of religion and spirituality, especially among the youth of Gen Z, Brent Potter brings a depth and clarify to the question of faith and its implications for our lives."

Brent Dean Robbins, Ph.D., *Program Director, Department of Psychology, Point Park University and Author of* The Medicalized Body and Anesthetic Culture: The Cadaver, the Memorial Body, and the Recovery of Lived Experience

Elements of Faith: Psychoanalytic Phenomenon and Lived Experience

Global Literature and the Environment analyses literatures from across the world that connect readers to the localized impacts of the climate and ecological emergencies. The book contextualizes ecological breakdown within the history of capitalist-imperialism, exploring how literature helps us to imagine and create a habitable and just world for all forms of life.

The four chapters are organized according to the elements of the climate system that are at risk. 'Earth' examines Caribbean, American, South African, and British literatures that explore how dominant human groups have exploited soils, minerals, metals, and oil in pursuit of economic aims. 'Water' engages with poetic representations of, and responses to, extraction, pollution, and global warming in the fresh- and saltwaters of Nigeria and the icescapes of Alaska. 'Air' analyses prose and poetry that depicts atmospheric pollution caused by gas flaring in the Niger Delta and the production of pesticides in India. 'Life' attends to the ways in which literature contextualizes the drivers of, and proposed solutions to, mass species extinction across North America, Africa, Australasia, and Aotearoa New Zealand.

This accessible and engaging book explores novels, plays, and poetry by writers including Octavia Butler, C.L.R. James, dg nanouk okpik, Ken Saro-Wiwa, Imbolo Mbue, Indra Sinha, Witi Ihimaera, J.M. Coetzee, and Henrietta Rose-Innes, amongst many others. It introduces readers to the concept of the Anthropocene alongside perspectives that challenge the assumption that the climate crisis is caused by an undifferentiated humanity. In doing so, the book draws on, and combines, a range of theoretical approaches, including postcolonialism, Indigenous studies, ecocriticism, cultural materialism, and animal studies.

Brent Potter is a psychoanalyst and author known for his work at the intersection of psychology, philosophy, and faith. With over three decades of clinical experience, his writing explores the depths of human suffering, healing, and meaning through accessible yet profound existential and psychoanalytic inquiry.

Routledge Focus on Mental Health

Routledge Focus on Mental Health presents short books on current topics, linking in with cutting-edge research and practice.

Efficient Therapy for Specific Client Problems
Making the Most of Every Client Session
Windy Dryden

The Mind of Complex Numbers and the Subject in Analyses
Raul Moncayo

Being a Crisis Chaplain
Delivering Help and Healing in Critical Scenarios
Sidney Dekker and Lance Mergard

A Critical Examination of Irvin D. Yalom's Single Session Consultations
It Is the Relationship That Heals
Windy Dryden

The Power of Being a Subject
Transcending Human Mechanics with Critical Thinking, Honesty, Patience, and Bravery
Matthew H. Bowker

The Knowledge of the Psychoanalyst
Raul Moncayo

Elements of Faith: Psychoanalytic Phenomenon and Lived Experience
Brent Potter

For more information about this series, please visit: www.routledge.com/Routledge-Focus-on-Mental-Health/book-series/RFMH

Elements of Faith: Psychoanalytic Phenomenon and Lived Experience

Brent Potter

Routledge
Taylor & Francis Group
LONDON AND NEW YORK

First published 2026
by Routledge
4 Park Square, Milton Park, Abingdon, Oxon OX14 4RN

and by Routledge
605 Third Avenue, New York, NY 10158

Routledge is an imprint of the Taylor & Francis Group, an Informa business

British Library Cataloguing in Publication Data
A catalogue record for this book is available from the British Library

ISBN: 978-1-041-09982-6 (hbk)
ISBN: 978-1-041-10072-0 (pbk)
ISBN: 978-1-003-65321-9 (ebk)

DOI: 10.4324/9781003653219

Typeset in Times New Roman
by Taylor & Francis Books

Contents

To my wife, Gene Rose – my *Marilag*,
whose present and unseen acts of love and strength
have carried me and our children in more ways than can be measured.

Thank you for walking beside me with clarity, loving kindness, and grit.

Mahal po kita.

Acknowledgements

My heartfelt gratitude goes to my mentors—Ron Shaffer, Brent Dean Robbins, and Mike Eigen. Beyond their generous and abundant guidance, these men have modeled something even greater: how to be a better person. For that, I am especially grateful.

To the teachers who went above and beyond in offering wisdom and direction—Daniel Burston, Michael Sipiora, James Grotstein, Avedis Panajian, Kathy Rives, Lionel Corbett, James Hillman, Richard Capobianco, Robert Romanyshyn, and Richard Tarnas—thank you for shaping both my thought and my path.

To my past analysts and supervisors — Corwin Fergus, Lew Barth, Joye Weisel-Barth, George Bermudez, James Grotstein, and Avedis Panajian — thank you for guiding me through the uncharted places, and for helping me learn to read the landscape for myself.

1 Echoes of an Opening

Introductory Comments

This volume builds upon my earlier works, *Elements of Self-Destruction* (Potter, 2018a) and *Elements of Reparation: Truth, Faith, and Transformation in the Works of Heidegger, Bion, and Beyond* (Potter, 2018b), extending the exploration of faith as a multifaceted phenomenon. Here, I weave together reflections on faith with an intimate portrayal of my therapeutic journey with Sara, illustrating her transformation through our psychoanalytic collaboration.

The text integrates insights from psychoanalytic and phenomenological literature on faith, blending a comprehensive literature review with a detailed analytic case study. This thematic hermeneutic approach emphasizes the dynamic interplay between theory and practice, merging historical context with the immediacy of lived experience. By engaging with the past through psychoanalytic theory and anchoring it in the present through praxis, the work reveals a "fusion of horizons." This synthesis allows faith to emerge as a resonant phenomenon, bridging intellectual understanding and emotional depth and enriching both theoretical and practical dimensions of psychoanalytic inquiry.

Faith Fragments

Faith is, at once, one of the most enigmatic and essential dimensions of human life. It is a phenomenon that has shaped civilizations and unsettled philosophers, stirred the hearts of the faithful and eluded the grasp of the skeptic. Rooted in conviction and longing, faith transcends the confines of doctrine and ritual; it is not reducible to belief alone, but emerges as a profound human orientation – one that seeks meaning amidst the uncertainty of existence.

DOI: 10.4324/9781003653219-1

What follows is not an exhaustive phenomenology of faith. No single text could contain so vast and elusive a subject. Instead, I offer fragments – glimpses of faith's many faces – alongside a psychoanalytic inquiry, culminating in a clinical case study. These fragments do not presume to map the entirety of faith's terrain, but rather gesture toward its contours, inviting the reader into a dialogue with something far larger than what can be summarized.

Life lives in faith; faith permeates life, every single cell. That does not exclude faithlessness, no-faith, and the empty bottom.

And psychoanalytic faith? The work of faith in sessions?

…many sessions are crises of faith. Is life worth living? With what quality? How? Or is a soul too crippled to go on, too infected with ill spirit? (Eigen, 2014 , p. xii)

Across times and cultures, faith has remained a steady, if quiet, presence in the human story. From the star-watchers of the ancient world to the theologians and analysts of modernity, faith has shaped humanity's highest hopes and deepest questions. Whether expressed in public devotion, philosophical reflection, or the private convictions that carry life forward, faith endures because it addresses something essential: the space between what is and what might be, between what we know and what we long for.

This inquiry proceeds from the recognition that faith cannot be confined to the precincts of religion or reduced to an intellectual assent. Faith, in its most elemental form, is an existential phenomenon – a structure of experience that carries with it trust, hope, and a wager on the unseen. It arises precisely where certainty fails; it begins where proof ends. And yet, it is no less real for its refusal to submit to verification.

To speak of faith is also to speak of its complexity. It is a phenomenon braided from multiple strands – psychological, philosophical, cultural, and theological. Faith informs identities and ethical commitments; it bears upon political landscapes and personal reckonings alike. It can console and divide, liberate and constrain. Any serious consideration of faith must therefore engage its paradoxes and tensions, refusing the temptation to resolve them too quickly.

In the pages that follow, we will traverse these complexities. We will examine faith not as an abstraction, but as a lived, embodied phenomenon – one that emerges in moments of anguish and awe, in the clinical encounter, and in the everyday labor of making meaning. Through analytic reflection and clinical illustration, we will trace faith's contours and contradictions, illuminating its presence not only in the grand narratives of religion and philosophy, but also in the quiet corners of human experience.

Navigating the Landscape

As we embark on an exploration of faith, it is important to approach this journey with an open and respectful mindset, recognizing the sensitivity and personal significance these subject holds for many. Faith, in its myriad forms, transcends boundaries of culture, religion, and philosophy, serving as both a deeply personal experience and a collective phenomenon. Our intent is not to advocate for or challenge any particular belief system but rather to engage in a thoughtful and holistic analysis of faith itself – its essence, its manifestations, and its impact on the human condition. By adopting this inclusive and reflective stance, we aim to honor the diversity of perspectives and experiences that faith encompasses, acknowledging its power to inspire, comfort, challenge, and transform.

Faith is a phenomenon that has shaped human history, ignited debates, and stirred the depths of the human soul for millennia. It is a force that transcends time, geography, and ideology, uniting people in a shared purpose while simultaneously provoking profound questions about existence, meaning, and the nature of the universe. To understand faith is to delve into the intricate tapestry of beliefs, doubts, hopes, and fears that constitute the foundation of human experience. It invites us to examine the ways in which individuals and communities navigate the mysteries of life, grapple with uncertainty, and find meaning in the face of the unknown.

In the chapters that follow, we will embark on a multidimensional exploration of faith, examining its psychological, philosophical, cultural, and existential dimensions. We will consider how faith operates within the human psyche, shaping identity, guiding behavior, and influencing relationships. From a philosophical perspective, we will delve into the questions of truth, belief, and knowledge that faith evokes, exploring its intersections with reason and intuition. Culturally, we will examine how faith traditions have evolved, adapted, and interacted with one another, leaving indelible marks on art, literature, and social structures. Existentially, we will reflect on the ways faith provides solace and purpose in the face of life's uncertainties, offering a framework for navigating the complexities of existence.

This journey of understanding is not merely an intellectual endeavor but an invitation to introspection and dialogue. It calls upon us to set aside preconceived notions and engage with the phenomenon of faith on its own terms, appreciating its nuances and contradictions. Through this process, we aim to uncover the layers of meaning that faith embodies, recognizing its capacity to inspire both profound devotion and critical inquiry.

As we lay the groundwork for this exploration, we invite readers to join us in contemplating the essence of faith and its profound influence on the intricate mosaic of humanity. This introduction serves as a guidepost, setting the stage for the chapters to come and highlighting the significance, complexity, and multifaceted nature of faith. We begin this inquiry with the hope of shedding light, however partially, on the enduring mystery of faith and its role in human being.

2 Dimensions of Faith

At the heart of human experience lies a phenomenon both fundamental and transcendent: faith. This chapter takes up the task of examining faith's nature, tracing the intricate web of beliefs, convictions, and intuitions that give shape to this defining aspect of human life. In its many forms and expressions, faith stands as a source of hope, a wellspring of meaning, and a lens through which individuals make sense of the complexities of existence.

Faith's essence resides in its ability to transcend the boundaries of empirical evidence and rational comprehension. It embodies a belief in something intangible, an unwavering trust in truths that extend beyond immediate sensory experiences. Faith often leads individuals to embrace concepts, ideas, or entities that exist beyond the grasp of the physical world. Whether directed toward a higher power, a philosophical doctrine, or the potential for personal growth, faith serves as a bridge between the known and the unknown, the seen and the unseen.

Belief stands as a cornerstone of faith, forming the foundation upon which the experience of faith is built. At its core, belief is more than the intellectual acknowledgment of a concept or proposition; it is an intricate interplay of cognition, emotion, and conviction. It involves the acceptance of ideas or principles as truth, but also the emotional resonance and personal significance that give those ideas their power. Belief is not merely a passive state of mind; it is an active engagement with the world, a lens through which individuals interpret their experiences and derive meaning.

The essence of faith is inextricably linked to the transformative power of belief. It is belief that gives faith its vitality, enabling it to shape attitudes, behaviors, and perceptions in profound ways. When individuals hold a belief with conviction, it becomes a driving force that influences their choices and actions, guiding them toward goals

DOI: 10.4324/9781003653219-2

and values that align with their faith. This dynamic relationship between belief and faith underscores how deeply personal and impactful faith can be, as it motivates people to transcend their limitations, persevere through challenges, and pursue aspirations that reflect their innermost values.

Belief operates on multiple levels, encompassing both conscious and unconscious dimensions. On one hand, it involves deliberate reflection and rational consideration as individuals evaluate the validity and implications of their beliefs. On the other hand, belief is also shaped by emotional and psychological factors, including trust, hope, and a sense of connection to something greater than oneself. This duality highlights the complexity of belief, as it is influenced by both reason and emotion, intellect, and intuition.

Through belief, faith becomes a dynamic and active force in a person's life, manifesting in thoughts, words, and deeds. It is through belief that faith inspires individuals to commit to causes, engage in practices, and cultivate relationships that reflect their values and convictions. Belief provides the framework within which faith can flourish, offering a sense of purpose and direction that empowers individuals to navigate life's uncertainties with confidence and resolve.

Moreover, belief has the power to shape perceptions, influencing how individuals interpret the world around them. It colors their understanding of events, relationships, and experiences, imbuing them with meaning and significance. This interpretive function of belief underscores its role in shaping not only individual attitudes but also collective identities and cultural narratives. Through shared beliefs, communities come together, finding common ground and fostering a sense of belonging that strengthens their faith.

In a sense, belief is the engine that drives faith, transforming abstract principles into lived experiences. It propels individuals to act in alignment with their convictions, investing themselves in pursuits that resonate with their faith. Whether expressed through acts of kindness, creative endeavors, or steadfast commitment to ideals, belief gives faith its tangible expression, allowing it to influence the world in meaningful and enduring ways. By examining the multifaceted nature of belief, we gain a deeper appreciation for its central role in the phenomenon of faith and its profound impact on human experience.

While faith is often associated with unwavering conviction, it is not immune to doubt and uncertainty. In fact, the interplay between doubt and faith can serve as a catalyst for deeper introspection and spiritual growth. The essence of faith extends beyond blind acceptance; it thrives on the tension between doubt and conviction, inviting individuals to engage in critical reflection, seek understanding, and ultimately arrive at a place of steadfast belief.

Emotions play a profound role in shaping the essence of faith. The feelings evoked by faith are as diverse as the belief systems they underpin. From the serenity of trust to the enthusiasm of devotion, the emotional dimensions of faith encompass everything from inner peace to passionate dedication. Faith can provide solace in times of adversity, inspire acts of compassion, and kindle the flame of hope when circumstances seem bleak. It is this emotional undercurrent that infuses faith with vitality, making it a deeply personal and transformative experience.

Faith's essence is closely tied to the recognition that human understanding has its limits and that truths exist beyond rational comprehension. It prompts individuals to venture into the realms of the mysterious and the metaphysical, where the heart and spirit find resonance even in the absence of tangible evidence. Faith invites individuals to explore the uncharted territories of meaning, purpose, and existential significance that lie beyond empirical observation.

In tracing the essence of faith, we encounter a phenomenon that defies easy categorization and encapsulates the intricacies of human belief, trust, and conviction. Faith reaches deep into the human psyche, inspiring courage in the face of uncertainty, fostering empathy and compassion, and providing a lens through which to perceive the wonders of the world. Through faith, individuals navigate the complexities of life, drawing upon the power of belief and recognizing truths that extend beyond the visible horizon.

As a potent force that shapes human beliefs and behaviors, faith finds its most profound and varied expressions within the tapestry of religious traditions. This chapter embarks on a captivating journey through the intricate relationship between faith and religion, exploring how faith becomes the lifeblood of the rituals, doctrines, and practices that give structure to the spiritual lives of millions.

The Role of Sacred Texts: Anchors of Faith

Faith may be understood as the soul's memory of God – a deep, often unspoken awareness of something beyond the visible world. Within the fabric of religious traditions, sacred texts hold a central place. These writings are not merely literary artifacts; they are vessels of wisdom, moral instruction, and historical memory that ground and sustain the faith of their communities. Whether the Torah, the Quran, the Bhagavad Gita, or the Bible, such texts serve as more than repositories of doctrine – they act as bridges between the human and the divine, carrying faith across generations and nurturing a living connection between individuals and the sacred. Religious doctrines and dogmas form the bedrock upon which faith is built within religious communities. This section explores how these belief systems provide a framework for understanding the nature of the divine, the purpose of existence, and the ethical codes that guide human conduct. From the Trinity in Christianity to the Four Noble Truths in Buddhism, these core tenets shape the contours of faith, guiding believers on their spiritual journeys and offering a sense of unity and purpose.

Central to faith in religious traditions are the rituals and practices that facilitate a connection with the divine. Through prayer, meditation, fasting, or pilgrimage, these rituals serve as powerful expressions of devotion, allowing believers to seek solace and engage in communion with the sacred. This section explores the multifaceted nature of religious traditions, their significance in deepening faith, and their ability to foster a sense of community among believers.

Within religious traditions, faith often extends beyond the boundaries of rationality, leading individuals to explore the mystical dimensions of existence. Mysticism, with its emphasis on direct experiences of the divine or transcendent, offers a unique perspective on faith's essence. This section delves into the mystical undercurrents of faith, highlighting practices such as Sufi whirling, Christian contemplative prayer, and Hindu meditation, which provide believers with glimpses of the ineffable and foster a profound sense of connection to the divine.

The communal aspect of faith is vividly exemplified within religious congregations and institutions. This section examines how faith thrives in collective worship, shared rituals, and the fellowship of believers. It discusses the role of religious leaders – such as priests, imams, rabbis, and gurus – who guide and nourish the faith of their congregants. Additionally, the impact of faith-based communities on shaping cultural identity, providing social support, and contributing to broader society is explored.

Faith, as nurtured within religious traditions, often serves as a moral compass that informs ethical choices and behavior. This section examines how religious teachings and faith-based values influence individuals' decisions, shaping their interactions with others and their contributions to the world. It explores how faith-driven moral imperatives inspire acts of compassion, justice, and social responsibility, reinforcing the notion that faith extends beyond personal belief to impact the larger human community.

The exploration of faith within religious traditions unveils a world rich in symbolism, devotion, and shared meaning. These traditions provide individuals with a framework to navigate life's complexities, offering solace, guidance, and a sense of belonging. By examining how faith finds expression within religious contexts, we gain insights into the transformative power of belief, the intricacies of worship, and the role of communal practices in nurturing a profound and enduring connection to the divine.

As an intricate tapestry woven through human experience, faith also finds a compelling presence within the realm of philosophy. This chapter embarks on a journey through the philosophical landscape of faith, where reason and belief intersect, existential questions arise, and the boundaries of human understanding are pushed to their limits. From the existential leaps of faith to the debates surrounding reason and belief, we delve into the philosophical inquiries that have shaped our understanding of this complex phenomenon.

Faith and Reason: A Delicate Balance

The interplay between faith and reason has occupied a prominent position in philosophical discourse for centuries, reflecting humanity's enduring quest to reconcile the spiritual and the rational. These two intellectual forces, often perceived as opposing, have sparked debates that delve into the very nature of belief, truth, and understanding. This section traces the evolution of thought surrounding this dynamic relationship, beginning with the medieval scholastics who sought to harmonize faith with reason and continuing through the Enlightenment thinkers who championed critical inquiry and empirical evidence.

Medieval philosophers such as Thomas Aquinas epitomized the effort to bridge faith and reason, arguing that the two are not inherently contradictory but complementary. Aquinas maintained that reason could lead to an understanding of certain truths about the divine, while faith provided access to mysteries beyond human comprehension. His work, along with that of other scholastics, established a framework in which faith and reason were seen as distinct yet mutually reinforcing pathways to truth. This synthesis of theology and philosophy underscored the belief that rational thought could serve as a tool to deepen one's understanding of faith.

The Enlightenment, however, brought a shift in perspective. Thinkers such as Immanuel Kant and David Hume emphasized the primacy of reason and empirical evidence, often challenging traditional religious doctrines. This era saw a growing tension between faith's reliance on transcendent truths and reason's demand for critical inquiry and verifiable knowledge. Yet, even in this age of rationalism, some philosophers sought to explore the possibility of coexistence. Kant, for instance, proposed that while reason could not fully comprehend the divine, it could provide a moral foundation that resonated with religious principles, suggesting a potential harmony between the two.

In contemporary discourse, the tension between faith and reason continues to inspire exploration. The ability of faith to transcend empirical evidence and engage with the ineffable contrasts with reason's insistence on logical consistency and factual validation. However, these faculties need not be seen as irreconcilable. When faith and reason coexist, they can create a richer, more nuanced understanding of the world. Faith can inspire purpose and hope, while reason provides the tools for critical analysis and practical application. Together, they offer a holistic approach to navigating the complexities of human existence.

Existentialist philosophy invites us to confront profound questions about existence, purpose, and the human condition, often placing faith at the center of these inquiries. This section examines the contributions of existentialist thinkers such as Søren Kierkegaard, Friedrich Nietzsche, Jean-Paul Sartre, and Albert Camus, whose writings grapple with the role of faith in a universe that frequently appears indifferent or absurd.

Kierkegaard, often regarded as the father of existentialism, introduced the concept of the "leap of faith." He argued that faith requires an individual to embrace uncertainty and take a personal, subjective leap beyond the limits of reason. For Kierkegaard, this leap was not a rejection of rationality but an acknowledgment of its boundaries. Faith, in his view, was a deeply personal act of trust in the face of existential doubt, a means of finding meaning in a world that often defies explanation.

Nietzsche, in contrast, challenged traditional notions of faith, famously declaring the "death of God" and urging humanity to create its own values in the absence of divine authority. His critique of religious faith was not merely a rejection but a call to confront the existential implications of a godless universe. Nietzsche's work underscores the tension between faith and reason, highlighting the struggle to find meaning and purpose in a world devoid of inherent order.

Sartre and Camus further expanded on these themes, exploring the implications of human freedom and the absurdity of existence. Sartre's concept of the "anguish of freedom" emphasized the weight of responsibility that comes with the realization that individuals are free to define their own existence. This freedom, while liberating, also engenders a profound sense of existential anxiety. Camus, on the other hand, grappled with the "absurd," the conflict between humanity's desire for meaning and the universe's apparent indifference. In works such as *The Myth of Sisyphus*, Camus (2018) suggested that faith might offer solace, but he ultimately advocated for embracing the absurd and finding meaning through human resilience and creativity.

These existentialist perspectives challenge individuals to face the dilemmas that faith seeks to address, urging a deeper engagement with questions of meaning, purpose, and authenticity. By exploring the interplay between faith and reason, as well as the existential dimensions of belief, we gain insight into the complexities of the human experience. This examination reveals that faith, far from being a simple or static concept, is a dynamic force that interacts with reason, culture, and individual choice, shaping the ways in which we navigate the profound mysteries of existence.

Faith and Ethics: A Moral Framework

Within the philosophical realm, faith significantly shapes ethical frameworks and guides moral decisions. This section delves into how faith contributes to discussions on moral absolutism, relativism, and the foundations of ethical behavior. We examine how faith-based belief systems provide individuals with moral grounding, influencing their judgments, actions, and interactions with others. Additionally, we consider the challenges and ethical dilemmas that may arise when faith-driven convictions clash with broader societal values.

At the heart of philosophical inquiry lies the timeless quest for meaning and purpose. This section explores how faith serves as a response to the existential vacuum, offering individuals narratives that imbue life with significance and direction. We delve into Viktor Frankl's (2006, 2019, 2021) existential analysis and his assertion that faith contributes to a sense of meaning even in the face of suffering. This exploration extends to how faith provides a framework for navigating the complexities of human existence and finding purpose within a chaotic world.

Epistemology, the branch of philosophy concerned with knowledge and belief, offers insights into the complexities of faith as a form of belief. This section examines the works of philosophers such as William James (2018), who explored the subjective nature of religious experience, and Thomas Aquinas (1997), who investigated the relationship between faith and reason. We consider the concept of "justified belief" and how faith's validity is assessed within different epistemological frameworks, shedding light on how faith can coexist with rational inquiry.

The philosophical exploration of faith invites us to traverse the realms of reason, existential contemplation, and ethical inquiry. From the delicate balance between faith and reason to existentialist confrontations with meaninglessness, philosophy provides a platform for grappling with the profound questions that faith seeks to address. As we navigate the philosophical landscape of faith, we gain a deeper appreciation for the nuanced interplay between belief and reason and the enduring quest to reconcile the mysteries of existence with the limits of human understanding.

Amid the intricate tapestry of human experience, the threads of faith and identity are interwoven in ways that shape personal and collective narratives. This section embarks on a journey through the complex relationship between faith and identity, examining how beliefs influence self-perception, cultural affiliation, and individuals' engagement with the world around them. From the formation of cultural identity to the role of faith in shaping individual uniqueness, we explore the dynamic interplay between these two fundamental aspects of human existence.

Cultural identity is often intricately intertwined with faith, serving as a defining marker for individuals and communities. This section explores how faith contributes to the formation of cultural identities, reflecting the values, traditions, and worldviews of specific groups. We delve into the ways religious practices, rituals, and symbols become integral to cultural expression, providing a sense of continuity and belonging that transcends generations. By examining how faith informs cultural identity, we gain insight into the powerful connections that bind individuals to their heritage and community.

Religious faith serves as a unique lens through which individuals perceive the world and navigate their surroundings. This section investigates how faith shapes perspectives, influences decision-making, and impacts interactions with others. We explore how religious narratives, teachings, and moral codes provide a framework for understanding societal norms and values. By examining the interplay between faith and cultural interpretation, we uncover the intricate ways in which belief systems contribute to the construction of both individual and collective worldviews.

Faith communities – whether religious congregations, spiritual groups, or philosophical circles – act as crucibles for cultivating social bonds and shared identities. This section delves into the role of faith-based communities in fostering belonging, support, and mutual understanding among their members. We explore the rituals, gatherings, and collaborative efforts that solidify connections within these communities. Additionally, we examine how faith-driven social initiatives and charitable endeavors extend the formation of identity beyond individual beliefs.

Beyond cultural and communal dimensions, faith plays a pivotal role in shaping individual identities. This section explores how personal beliefs influence self-perception, aspirations, and life choices. We examine how faith provides a source of meaning and purpose, contributing to the development of a unique and authentic identity. Whether through religious vocation, spiritual exploration, or adherence to philosophical tenets, faith becomes an integral part of the narrative individuals construct about themselves.

The Hebraic Mindset: A Necessary Counterbalance

While the Greek philosophical tradition has heavily influenced Western theology and psychology – with its emphasis on abstraction, essence, and static being – the Hebraic worldview offers an essential and often overlooked corrective: a lived, relational, embodied faith grounded in history, action, and covenant.

Whereas Greek thought often prioritizes ontology (what something is), Hebraic consciousness is oriented around function and relationship. To be is not merely to exist but to act, to participate, to respond. In this frame, faith (*emunah*) is not assent to propositions but fidelity in relationship – a trust lived out, rather than believed in the abstract. Likewise, righteousness (*tsedaqah*) is not an interior moral quality alone but right-relatedness in context: to neighbor, to God, to the earth.

This mode of thought resists the split between mind and body, theory and practice, sacred and secular. It also offers a profound psychological insight: transformation does not arise from intellectual comprehension alone, but from participation in a shared narrative. We are not saved by ideas; we are saved in time, in place, in flesh.

The therapeutic implications of this are immense. In the Hebraic view, healing does not occur outside of history. The analysand is not a detached psyche but a storied being – a person whose wounds and hope are embedded in their familial, cultural, and spiritual inheritance. The clinical space becomes a kind of covenantal encounter: not a transaction, but a relationship sustained by presence, memory, and promise.

This contrasts with the more atomized individual so often assumed in modern psychology – a disembodied self navigating a world of techniques. The Hebraic frame restores the person to the field of belonging. It says: You are not alone. You are not reducible to your symptoms. You are part of a people, a promise, a pilgrimage.

Bringing this to bear on *Elements of Faith*, the Hebraic consciousness joins the existential-phenomenological and psychoanalytic traditions by insisting that the deepest truths are not only felt inwardly, but enacted communally. The self is not isolated. It is summoned.

Here, the goal of psychoanalytic inquiry is not simply insight but return – to one's face, one's name, one's inheritance. And ultimately, to one's God.

This is not an argument for abandoning Greek categories, but for recovering the Hebraic pulse beneath them. Together, they form a dialectic that makes *Elements of Faith* whole: a faith that is thought and lived, analyzed and embodied, crucified and resurrected.

3 Faith in a Pluralistic World

Contours of Disruption: Faith Amid the They

The interplay between faith and identity is a nuanced and multifaceted dynamic deeply embedded in the fabric of human existence. It is not without its challenges, particularly in a world increasingly characterized by cultural diversity, globalization, and the rapid intermingling of traditions, beliefs, and worldviews. Faith, as a deeply personal yet inherently communal phenomenon, profoundly influences how individuals perceive themselves and how they relate to their broader society. At the same time, identity, shaped by cultural affiliations, historical contexts, and personal experiences, serves as a lens through which faith is understood and expressed. Together, these forces create a complex, ever-evolving relationship that is as enriching as it is challenging.

In multicultural societies, the intersection of differing belief systems often highlights the tensions that arise from religious pluralism. On the one hand, pluralism reflects the richness of human diversity, offering opportunities for dialogue, learning, and mutual enrichment. On the other hand, it can also give rise to misunderstandings, prejudice, and conflict, particularly when faith-based identities are perceived as incompatible or threatening to one another. These tensions are often amplified in the context of globalization, where the rapid exchange of ideas and cultural practices can blur traditional boundaries and challenge established norms. Faith, as a core component of identity, may be both a source of resilience and a point of contention as individuals and communities navigate the complexities of coexistence in an interconnected world.

Religious pluralism, while a testament to humanity's diversity, demands careful negotiation to foster harmony and understanding. The coexistence of multiple faith traditions within a single society

DOI: 10.4324/9781003653219-3

requires not only tolerance but also a commitment to genuine engagement and respect. Interfaith dialogue emerges as a crucial tool in this endeavor, providing a platform for individuals and communities to share their beliefs, address misconceptions, and build bridges of understanding. Through dialogue, differences can be acknowledged without eroding the unique identities that faith imparts, creating a foundation for peaceful coexistence and mutual respect. Such efforts are vital in countering the polarization and divisiveness that can arise when faith-based identities are weaponized or misunderstood.

The challenges posed by the interplay of faith and identity are not limited to external conflicts; they also manifest within individuals as they navigate the tensions between personal beliefs, cultural expectations, and societal norms. Faith often serves as a guiding force, offering a sense of purpose, moral grounding, and connection to a larger narrative. Yet, it can also be a source of internal struggle, particularly when personal convictions conflict with the expectations of one's cultural or social environment. These struggles highlight the deeply personal nature of faith and its role in shaping individual identity, as well as the broader cultural dynamics that influence how faith is lived and expressed.

Faith communities play a pivotal role in this interplay, serving as spaces where individuals find support, belonging, and opportunities for collective expression. These communities often act as custodians of tradition, preserving and transmitting the values, rituals, and narratives that define a particular faith. At the same time, they are also sites of negotiation and adaptation, where members grapple with the challenges of maintaining their identity in a rapidly changing world. By fostering social bonds and providing a sense of shared purpose, faith communities contribute to the formation of cultural identities and the weaving of individual experiences into the broader fabric of human existence.

Exploring the relationship between faith and identity reveals a rich and complex tapestry that reflects the diverse and interconnected nature of the human experience. It invites us to consider how faith shapes individual uniqueness, offering a profound sense of meaning and purpose while also contributing to collective belonging and cultural continuity. By delving into this intricate interplay, we gain a deeper appreciation of the ways in which faith and identity coexist, sometimes in harmony, sometimes in tension, but always as integral components of the human story. In confronting the challenges that arise from this relationship, we open the door to a more inclusive and empathetic understanding of ourselves and the world we share.

Faith as a Catalyst for Change

"Men stumble over pebbles, never over mountains" (Cady, 2014, p. 51). Embedded within the human spirit, faith possesses the remarkable power to inspire transformation and catalyze change on individual, societal, and global scales. This chapter explores the dynamic role that faith plays as a catalyst for change, examining how beliefs, convictions, and spiritual insights propel individuals and communities to challenge norms, advocate for justice, and contribute to the betterment of the world around them.

Faith has historically served as a driving force behind social movements and advocacy efforts aimed at fostering positive change. This section examines how religious and spiritual convictions have fueled movements for civil rights, gender equality, environmental sustainability, and humanitarian aid. We explore how faith provides individuals with the moral imperative to address societal injustices and advocate for the rights and dignity of marginalized populations. By delving into the stories of faith-inspired activists, we uncover the transformative potential of belief to ignite movements that challenge the status quo.

Faith often serves as a moral compass, guiding individuals toward acts of compassion and altruism. This section explores how faith-based values inspire believers to engage in charitable endeavors, contribute to community well-being, and extend a helping hand to those in need. By examining faith-driven initiatives, we gain insight into how belief systems motivate selfless acts of service that enrich lives, uplift communities, and exemplify the transformative power of faith in action.

Religious institutions, as pillars of faith, wield significant influence in shaping societal norms and values. This section examines how faith-based organizations contribute to positive change through education, humanitarian aid, and advocacy. We delve into the ways religious leaders, congregations, and institutions leverage their influence to address social issues, promote inclusivity, and foster dialogue. By exploring their roles as agents of change, we uncover the meaningful impact that faith-based institutions can have on societal transformation.

In an era marked by environmental challenges, faith emerges as a catalyst for sustainability and environmental stewardship. This section investigates how different belief systems and spiritual traditions advocate for the protection of the Earth and the responsible use of its resources. We explore how faith-driven principles align with ecological consciousness, inspiring individuals to adopt sustainable practices, advocate for environmental policies, and safeguard the planet for future generations.

Beyond its impact on external realities, faith often catalyzes personal transformation and inner growth. This section delves into how faith-based practices – such as meditation, prayer, and self-reflection – contribute to self-awareness, emotional well-being, and personal development. We explore how faith provides individuals with a framework for cultivating virtues, practicing mindfulness, and nurturing a sense of purpose that transcends material pursuits.

In an increasingly interconnected world, faith has the potential to transcend boundaries and foster global cooperation. This section examines the roles of interfaith dialogue, ecumenical efforts, and faith-based diplomacy in promoting understanding, peace, and collaboration across diverse cultures and belief systems. By exploring faith-driven initiatives that transcend geopolitical divides, we gain insight into the unifying power of shared values and the potential for faith to bridge differences and contribute to a harmonious global community.

The exploration of faith as a catalyst for change reveals an intersection where belief, conviction, and compassionate action inspire transformation. From the activism of faith-inspired movements to the inner growth nurtured by spiritual practices, faith proves to be a potent force capable of shaping the world in profound ways. By delving into the multifaceted role of faith as a catalyst for change, we deepen our appreciation of the transformative potential within the human spirit, inviting us to envision a future in which belief serves as a beacon of hope and positive impact.

Storms of Meaning

Faith, as a deeply personal and profound phenomenon, exists at the intersection of individual conviction and collective experience, making it inherently susceptible to challenges and controversies. These arise from a variety of sources, including divergent perspectives, ethical dilemmas, and the multifaceted complexities of an increasingly interconnected and diverse world. The examination of these challenges reveals the intricate and evolving nature of faith as it navigates tensions within religious contexts, ethical debates, and the interplay between belief and modernity.

Religious pluralism, the coexistence of diverse belief systems within a shared societal framework, is one of the most significant challenges facing faith in the modern era. The intersection of different faith traditions often brings conflicting worldviews to the forefront, leading to misunderstandings, tensions, and, at times, outright conflict. These challenges are particularly pronounced in multicultural societies, where religious diversity is both a strength and a potential source of division. The coexistence of such diversity necessitates a commitment to interfaith dialogue, which serves as a bridge for fostering mutual understanding and respect. Through open communication and the pursuit of common ground, individuals and communities can navigate the complexities of religious diversity, recognizing shared values while respecting differences. This process not only mitigates conflict but also enriches the collective human experience, offering opportunities for growth, learning, and collaboration.

Faith also places individuals and communities at the center of ethical dilemmas, especially when deeply-held beliefs come into conflict with broader societal values or legal frameworks. These conflicts are particularly evident in areas such as reproductive rights, end-of-life decisions, and LGBTQ+ perspectives, where personal convictions often clash with evolving norms and policies. For instance, debates over abortion rights highlight the tension between religious beliefs about the sanctity of life and the rights of individuals to make autonomous decisions about their bodies. Similarly, discussions surrounding physician-assisted dying challenge faith-based perspectives on the sanctity of life and suffering against arguments for personal dignity and autonomy. LGBTQ+ rights present another significant area of contention as faith communities grapple with reconciling traditional doctrines with the growing recognition of equality and inclusivity. Navigating these dilemmas requires individuals and communities to engage in nuanced, empathetic discussions that balance personal convictions with ethical responsibilities in a diverse and evolving society.

The rise of secularism and the rapid expansion of scientific knowledge further complicate faith's role in the modern world. As rationalism, materialism, and empirical inquiry continue to shape contemporary thought, faith is often called upon to justify its place in a landscape increasingly defined by scientific advancements and secular values. This tension is not new; it echoes historical debates such as those surrounding Darwin's theory of evolution or the heliocentric model of the solar system. Yet, the challenges of modernity demand fresh responses from faith communities. Believers must grapple with shifting paradigms of truth and understanding, reconciling spiritual beliefs with the empirical realities of the modern age. At the same time, faith has the potential to offer perspectives that complement scientific inquiry, addressing existential questions that science alone cannot fully answer. By engaging in dialogue with secularism and science, faith can adapt to the changing landscape of modernity, finding relevance and resonance in an increasingly complex world.

Within faith communities themselves, the interpretation of sacred texts and religious doctrines often gives rise to internal debates and divisions. Differing readings of religious texts can lead to divergent beliefs and practices, creating a dynamic interplay between orthodoxy and heterodoxy. These debates are further complicated by the role of religious authorities, who serve as interpreters and gatekeepers of tradition. In some cases, disagreements over interpretation can fracture communities, leading to the formation of new denominations or movements. However, these internal debates also reflect the vitality of faith, as believers seek to understand and apply their traditions in ways that are meaningful and relevant to their lives. The challenge lies in maintaining unity within diversity, fostering an environment where multiple interpretations can coexist while preserving the core values that bind communities together.

Hicks (2004) argues that postmodernism is not simply an academic or cultural trend but a full-fledged philosophical revolt – a force as socially corrosive and intellectually regressive as religious extremism. Both postmodernism and religious fanaticism, though seemingly opposites, converge in their shared attack on the Enlightenment legacy: reason, individual autonomy, objective knowledge, and liberal democracy. For Hicks, postmodernism is the radical offspring of failed socialist and collectivist ambitions. It emerges not only from epistemological skepticism but from political despair – a movement born of the collapse of rational arguments for socialism and the disillusionment with Marxist utopias.

At its core, Hicks claims, postmodernism denies the possibility of objective truth and reasoned discourse. Foucault, Derrida, Lyotard, and Rorty – the principal architects of the movement – explicitly reject truth as a meaningful category. Reason, they argue, is not a universal human faculty but a mask for power, a Western, white, male imposition on other groups. In place of rational argument, postmodernism offers a politics of language, identity, and ressentiment. It trades in deconstruction, irony, and rhetorical manipulation, refusing to be held accountable to standards of evidence or coherence. As Hicks notes, postmodern thinkers often admit that their assertions are not "true" in any conventional sense – they are strategic, deployed to undermine dominant structures and destabilize received meaning.

Herein lies the comparison with religious extremism. Just as religious fundamentalists assert truths that transcend reason and are not subject to empirical verification, postmodernists reject the very idea of rational justification. Both camps exhibit dogmatic certainty without rational foundation. Where the extremist invokes divine revelation or sacred texts, the postmodernist invokes lived experience, systemic oppression, or group identity as unassailable authority. In both cases, disagreement is not a matter of argument but a threat to the moral order. Those who dissent are not wrong – they are heretical, oppressive, or unworthy of engagement.

Moreover, both postmodernism and religious extremism view the liberal democratic order with deep suspicion. Hicks shows how Enlightenment liberalism – grounded in individual rights, limited government, and the rule of law – is anathematized by postmodern theorists. For them, liberalism is merely a cloak for capitalism and patriarchy. Even science, once heralded as a tool of emancipation, is cast as an instrument of domination. Postmodern feminists such as MacKinnon and Dworkin claim that "neutral" language and "objective" reason perpetuate male power. Lyotard derides science as just another narrative – no more valid than indigenous mythologies or marginalized worldviews. This leveling of truth claims leads not to pluralism, Hicks warns, but to the annihilation of dialogue.

Like religious extremism, postmodernism replaces rational persuasion with ideological conformity. It demands not merely that we listen to marginalized voices, but that we suspend judgment and accept all knowledge as socially constructed. Hicks emphasizes how this shift plays out in education, where the traditional aim of cultivating rational, independent thinkers is replaced by a commitment to social engineering. Students are no longer encouraged to seek truth or engage in rigorous inquiry; they are taught instead to affirm group identity, denounce systemic power, and view knowledge as a function of race, gender, and class.

Hicks traces this intellectual regression to the epistemological crisis inaugurated by Kant. Once reason was declared incapable of grasping noumenal reality, the door was opened to skepticism, relativism, and ultimately irrationalism. From Kant to Hegel, Nietzsche, Heidegger, and the postmoderns, Hicks charts a genealogy of ideas that systematically eroded confidence in reason, truth, and the individual. Simultaneously, he argues, the political Left – especially after the repeated failures of socialism in theory and practice – retreated from rational defense of its ideals. Postmodernism, then, became a refuge: a means of waging ideological warfare without having to justify claims in rational or empirical terms.

In Hicks's view, the danger of postmodernism lies in its cynical abandonment of truth as a cultural value. It does not offer an alternative vision of society grounded in shared ideals or universal principles. It offers instead a politics of fragmentation, perpetual grievance, and zero-sum conflict. Just as religious extremism reduces the complexity of the world to a binary of believers and infidels, postmodernism reduces all human interaction to oppressors and oppressed, truth-tellers and power brokers, the woke and the damned.

This ethos has real-world consequences. Hicks cites the politicization of the university, the erosion of liberal values, and the rise of speech codes, censorship, and ideological orthodoxy as signs of postmodernism's spread. Just as religious extremism seeks to purify society by silencing dissent, postmodernism uses the language of inclusion to exclude, the rhetoric of tolerance to punish, and the banner of justice to justify coercion.

Ultimately, Hicks calls for a return to Enlightenment principles – not as nostalgic dogma, but as the only viable framework for a pluralistic, democratic society. He urges defenders of reason, science, and liberty not to retreat but to reassert the moral and epistemological foundations of modernity. Like religious extremism, postmodernism cannot be negotiated with – it must be exposed and opposed at its roots.

The exploration of these challenges and controversies highlights the intricate relationship between faith and the world it inhabits. Faith is not a static or monolithic entity; it is a dynamic force that evolves in response to the complexities of human experience. By confronting these challenges with openness, humility, and a willingness to engage in dialogue, faith has the potential to transcend its limitations, offering solace, guidance, and transformative power to individuals and societies alike. In doing so, it reaffirms its relevance and resilience, even in the face of the profound uncertainties and contradictions of the modern age.

Faith and the Empirical Gaze

The relationship between faith and science has been a focal point of human inquiry for centuries, often marked by tension and debate. This tension arises primarily when scientific discoveries or theories appear to challenge long-held religious beliefs, creating a perceived dichotomy between faith-based and evidence-based ways of understanding the world. Historically, moments such as the Copernican revolution and Darwin's theory of evolution sparked significant conflicts, as they seemed to contradict the theological interpretations of the cosmos and human origins. These instances highlight the friction that can occur when faith and science operate in isolation, each asserting its own authority over questions of existence, purpose, and the nature of reality.

However, this narrative of conflict is not the full story. Throughout history, there have also been moments of harmony and mutual enrichment between faith and science. Many scientists, both past and present, have drawn inspiration from their faith, viewing their scientific endeavors as a means of exploring the divine order of creation. Figures such as Isaac Newton and Gregor Mendel exemplify how religious belief and scientific inquiry can coexist and even complement one another. Contemporary dialogues between theologians and scientists continue to bridge the gap, exploring questions about the origins of the universe, the nature of consciousness, and the ethical implications of technological advancements. By fostering constructive engagement, faith and science can work together to deepen humanity's understanding of the world, offering complementary perspectives that enrich the human experience.

Yet, while faith has the potential to inspire moral growth, compassion, and social progress, it is not immune to distortion. One of the most pressing challenges in the modern world is the rise of religious extremism, where radical interpretations of faith are used to justify violence, intolerance, and oppression. Extremism often arises from a combination of factors, including socio-political grievances, economic disparities, and a sense of cultural or religious alienation. These conditions create fertile ground for the manipulation of religious narratives to serve destructive agendas, leading to acts of terrorism, persecution, and the erosion of human rights.

The consequences of religious extremism and postmodernism (another religion, really) are far-reaching, affecting individuals, communities, and global stability. Violence fueled by radical ideologies undermines the core values of faith – love, compassion, and justice – replacing them with fear, hatred, and division. Efforts to combat extremism must address its root causes, such as poverty, marginalization, and lack of education, while also promoting interfaith dialogue, understanding, and the reinterpretation of religious texts in ways that emphasize their universal, life-affirming messages. Faith leaders, educators, and policymakers all have crucial roles to play in countering extremist ideologies while preserving the positive contributions of faith to society.

The exploration of these challenges underscores the intricate relationship between faith, societal dynamics, and ethical concerns. Faith, at its best, offers solace, guidance, and transformative power, shaping individuals and communities in profound ways. It can inspire acts of kindness, resilience in the face of adversity, and a sense of connection to something greater than oneself. However, faith must also navigate the complexities of a rapidly changing, pluralistic world. The global landscape demands that faith adapt to new realities, engaging with diverse perspectives and addressing pressing issues such as climate change, technological ethics, and social justice.

By confronting the challenges and controversies surrounding faith with honesty and openness, we gain a deeper appreciation for its multifaceted nature. Faith is neither static nor monolithic; it evolves in response to human experience, continually shaping and being shaped by the societies in which it exists. Through thoughtful dialogue, critical reflection, and a commitment to the values that unite humanity, faith can remain a powerful force for good, even in the face of the complexities and contradictions of the modern world. In this way, the relationship between faith and science, the fight against extremism, and the broader societal role of belief become part of a larger, ongoing conversation about what it means to be human in an ever-changing world.

4 Once, There Was a Longing…

Navigating the Boundaries of Faith

Before there is belief, there is ache. Longing precedes language, even the language of God. It stirs in the body like a hunger for something the world cannot name. In the earliest encounters of being – infancy's gaze, the trembling of trust, the mystery of the other – faith begins not as doctrine but as disposition. This disposition is a way of leaning toward the unknown, not in fear but in hopeful vulnerability.

In theological psychoanalysis, longing is not simply lack. It is a mode of attunement to being, a sensitivity to the "more" that always exceeds representation. Heidegger's notion of *Befindlichkeit* – our "foundness" in the world – suggests that moods disclose reality in a way that is more primordial than cognition. Longing, then, is not a symptom to be cured but a phenomenon to be listened to, held, and understood. It is the background music of the soul's theological life.

In clinical work, we often encounter those who mistake longing for failure. Clients may speak of emptiness, restlessness, the sense that "something is missing." Modern culture pathologizes this condition. The pharmaceutical and self-help industries alike promise to quieten the ache. But what if the ache is the most faithful part of us? What if faith begins not with knowing, but with staying – remaining with the ache long enough to allow it to speak?

To navigate the boundaries of faith is to make peace with this liminality. Faith is not static belief. It is a way of being-in-the-world that remains radically open. It is not reducible to certainty, but it is also not simply doubt. It is the space in which we are willing to be undone and reconstituted – not once, but again and again.

DOI: 10.4324/9781003653219-4

Roots on Fire: Faith Between Tradition and Change

We inherit more than eye color and surname. We inherit stories – cosmic, familial, ancestral. These stories root us. They give us rituals, rhythms, and roles. But they also constrict. Traditions, like the parental superego, can nourish or suffocate. As Winnicott reminds us, even a "good enough" tradition is one that allows for spontaneity and play.

Faith born in tradition is not passive. It must become one's own or wither into mimicry. There comes a time in every psychological and spiritual life when the root system must be disturbed. The soil may still be rich, but it must be loosened. The fire comes here – not to destroy, but to purify. This is the fire of individuation, of truth-seeking, of the refusal to reduce one's soul to inherited slogans.

We see this in adolescence, certainly, but also in midlife, in crisis, in grief. In these moments, the tradition that once held us may feel foreign. Laing described this rupture as a "breakthrough disguised as breakdown." Theologically, it may resemble the *dark night of the soul.* What psychoanalysis and theology share here is the refusal to foreclose meaning. The fire is not a sign of failure. It is often the beginning of the sacred becoming real.

To live faithfully between tradition and change is to become a liminal being – rooted but mobile, reverent but not rigid. The ego's task is not to eradicate tradition but to inhabit it authentically. Symbols must be reclaimed, not discarded. Rituals must be made real again. The tradition must become a dialogue, not a monologue.

Personal Belief and Collective Identity

Who we are is shaped by where we belong. Faith is never entirely private. It is learned in language, ritual, gaze. It is whispered by grandmothers, shouted in churches, embedded in gestures. Even those who disavow religion are responding to its presence.

Yet personal belief is not reducible to communal creed. The psychoanalytic journey is often a movement from identification to individuation – from "what they believe" to "what I know in my bones." This is not narcissism, but integration. The mature psyche holds both the need for community and the demand for truth.

Michael Eigen writes, "We need enough cohesion to stand being torn apart." Faith is this paradox. It unites us and isolates us. It calls us into communion and exile. To hold one's belief while remaining open to the faith of others is a mark of psychic maturity. It is not tolerance in the shallow sense, but reverence for the mystery of another's soul.

Collective identity can wound, especially when it demands conformity. But it can also heal when it reflects the diversity of voices within the self. The church, the temple, the mosque – each can become a holding environment or a psychic prison. The task is not to abandon them but to humanize them, to re-enter them as living beings rather than institutional artifacts.

The Evolution of Faith

Faith grows – but not always upward. Sometimes it retreats, doubles back, unravels. James Fowler offered a now-famous model of faith development, from the intuitive-projective stage of childhood to the universalizing faith of wisdom figures. Yet such models risk reducing the mystery to a staircase. Faith does not evolve in stages. It evolves in spirals, regressions, ruptures, and returns.

Psychoanalytically, faith mirrors the psyche: it splits, fragments, represses, mourns. But it also re-symbolizes, integrates, and surprises. The early faith that sought answers may evolve into a faith that lives the question, as Rilke encouraged. The God one prayed to in desperation may become the silence one learns to rest in.

This evolution is not toward more certainty, but deeper complexity. The ego learns that it cannot control God, the world, or even itself. And in that relinquishment, something freer arises – not submission, but surrender. A faith that has evolved is not a domesticated faith. It is a wild, living thing – ever on the edge of becoming.

Embracing the Mystery of Faith

Mystery is not a placeholder for ignorance. It is the ground from which faith springs. In theology, mystery is not absence but excess – the overflowing presence of the divine beyond conceptual grasp. In psychoanalysis, it is the unknowable within the self. The unconscious. The otherness of the other. The dream that escapes interpretation.

Faith that cannot tolerate mystery becomes dogma. It seeks to freeze the sacred into certainty. But as Bion teaches, thinking begins with not-knowing. The capacity to "remain in doubt without panic," as he puts it, is a precondition for psychic growth.

Michael Eigen writes beautifully of the "unknown God" within. Faith, he says, is not knowing what one believes but continuing to believe anyway. It is fidelity to the unseen. The psychoanalytic room, like the sanctuary, is a space where this fidelity is tested. Can we stay with the silence? Can we hear what we do not want to hear? Can we let go of the illusion that knowing is the same as being?

To embrace mystery is not to abandon thought, but to expand its horizon. Faith lives not beyond reason, but in a different register. A poetic register. A register of presence.

Faith, Sense, and Sensibility

Faith is not only a structure of thought. It is an orientation of feeling. It vibrates in the nerves, pulses in the chest. It is stirred by art, silence, music, poetry. It is moved by beauty and broken by grief. Faith is felt before it is known.

Merleau-Ponty reminds us that we do not perceive the world as detached observers but as embodied beings. Faith, then, is not an abstract assent. It is a sensuous engagement. It tastes, touches, trembles. It cries. It laughs. It dares to sing.

Sensibility is not sentimentality. It is the capacity to be moved. To be vulnerable to the world. To let the sacred in, not just through doctrine, but through the pores. A tree, a painting, a child's face – each may become a site of revelation.

Rilke wrote, "I want to be with those who know secret things or else alone." Faith is one of those secret things. Not secret because it is hidden, but because it cannot be explained. It must be lived. It must be sensed.

Faith is not a solution. It is a song. A sigh. A scent. A way of turning toward the world in love and terror and trembling hope.

5 A Clinical Case Study in Faith

Orientation to the Case Study

In this paper, I recount my psychoanalytic work with Sara, a case that brought the dynamics of *aphiemi* (forgiveness), faith, destructiveness, goodness, badness, stuckness, and *metanoia* (transformative change) into focus in poignant and meaningful ways. Capturing the full depth of this experience within a single paper is, of course, an impossibility. Yet I hope the reader will find a window into the shared qualitative space Sara and I occupied over our time together.

Author's Perspective and Bias

This work is presented as qualitative research in the form of a psychoanalytic case study. In qualitative research, acknowledging one's own perspectives and biases is essential (Fink, 2000). Therefore, before delving into Sara's story, I will briefly outline my background and perspective.

I am a middle-aged Caucasian male who has practiced clinical mental health for 30 years, during which I have maintained a private practice and held various organizational roles. Recognized as an expert in pediatric clinical issues and an ethnic minority mental health specialist (focused on African American and Native American populations) in Washington State, I began my educational journey with a bachelor's degree in research psychology from Western Washington University, followed by a master's in existential-phenomenological psychology from Duquesne University, and a PhD in Clinical Psychology from the Pacifica Graduate Institute with a concentration in depth psychology. Additionally, I hold doctorates in psychoanalysis: a PhD from Bircham University and a PsyD from the Institute for

DOI: 10.4324/9781003653219-5

Contemporary Psychoanalysis (ICP), where I also earned my certification to practice psychoanalysis.

As a practicing Christian, I have often attracted clients seeking cultural competency in this area. Currently, I work three 12-hour days, seeing 36 patients per week. My approach is rooted primarily in psychoanalysis, supplemented by Dialectical Behavioral Therapy (DBT) when appropriate. The intensive work I have undertaken over the last two years – both in supervision and my own analysis – has allowed me to deepen and apply my knowledge to my clinical practice. It was during this period that Sara came to me for counseling, drawn by my published work in Christian counseling and my experience with clients facing various forms of self-destructiveness.

At her intake, Sara received the same initial information I provide to all new clients. I explained my primary approach, which I describe as integrative relational psychoanalysis. Mitchell (1988) states that this perspective embraces different theories and traditions as enriching contributions to psychoanalytic practice, acknowledging both areas of compatibility and mutual exclusivity. My coursework, supervision, training analysis, and extensive experience over the years have helped shape this perspective. Specifically, it has allowed me to integrate research psychology, Jungian psychology, and Object Relations into a cohesive approach. My time at ICP was instrumental in synthesizing these perspectives and greatly enhanced my clinical capabilities. I found Mitchell's work especially resonant, providing an overarching framework that allowed me to draw upon my diverse training and background.

It's important to note that while I am informed by Mitchell, my practice is not an attempt to replicate his methods. Rather, I aim to hold my theoretical frameworks lightly, striving to follow the patient's lead, embrace vulnerability and unknowing, and allow myself to be moved by the patient, supporting them in finding a path forward (Orange, 2014).

Sara was informed of my affiliation with ICP, and in September 2020, we discussed the possibility of her becoming a control case. At that time, we met once or twice per week, but after she agreed to be a control case, our sessions increased to three or four times weekly. Sara understood and accepted that her case material might be used for my dissertation, embracing the opportunity for deeper, more intensive work.

All information about Sara in this paper has been carefully disguised to protect her anonymity, including her name. Her quotes are taken directly from her own writing and from my handwritten notes of her statements, ensuring their accuracy.

Sara: Patient Information Summary

Background

Sara, a middle-aged heterosexual Caucasian woman, first sought Christian counseling in the summer of 2020. She described struggling privately with symptoms of anxiety and depression for several years, compounded by the challenge of parenting adult children and reassessing her life. The immediate impetus for seeking help, however, was her youngest son's recent revelation that he is attracted to men. Sara, as a Christian, finds this revelation distressing and is concerned about his spiritual well-being. Although she has no history of mental health treatment, she values Christian counseling to align her mental health support with her faith.

Sara identifies culturally with her German heritage and conservative Lutheran background. Married for 39 years, she has two sons, aged 25 and 29. She has spent her career in healthcare, initially in nursing and now as an administrator overseeing physician education and training at a major university hospital. In addition to her demanding administrative role, she took on a contract as the lead COVID educator for her region.

Mental Health Symptoms and Concerns

Sara describes her depression and anxiety as pervasive, generalized affective states without specific triggers or acute episodes. She struggles to articulate the nature of her distress, instead referring to it as a constant "black 'blah' mass." Although Sara expresses concern over her depression, she is more focused on the implications of her son's sexuality, particularly fearing for his salvation.

Family and Relationships

Sara comes from a stable family with one younger sister and maintains close ties to her parents, who live nearby. Her relationship with her sister is strained, as they hold opposite views on various matters, including the COVID-19 pandemic. Despite their differences, Sara prioritizes family harmony, often suppressing her feelings to avoid conflict.

Sara reports no significant friendships or mentors from childhood to the present. Reflecting on her life, she explains that her focus has been on her career and family, leaving little time for other relationships. She describes her marriage as positive but notes that her husband, much like her father, is emotionally reserved. About 15 years ago, her husband suffered a work-related accident that resulted in chronic back pain, leading Sara to become the primary breadwinner, working long hours – often 90 to 100 hours per week – to support her family.

Coping and Boundaries

Sara describes herself as conflict-avoidant, often internalizing stress to keep the peace. She struggles with setting boundaries in her professional life, frequently overcommitting and finding it difficult to decline additional work projects. Her inability to say "no" at work has led to an absence of a healthy work-life balance, which she describes as "just the way life is."

Diagnostic Evaluation

In a collaborative approach to diagnosis, Sara and I discussed the possible diagnoses based on her symptoms and background. After reviewing her experiences and emotional landscape, we concluded that her symptoms aligned most closely with DSM-5 criteria for Persistent Depressive Disorder (300.4). Sara's depression appears to be pervasive rather than episodic, and her high level of functionality in various aspects of her life rules out Major Depressive Disorder. Although her background suggests potential sources of trauma, she does not meet the criteria for PTSD.

In exploring additional diagnostic context, McWilliams' (2011) psychoanalytic framework for depressive personalities provided further insight. Sara's symptoms align with McWilliams' description of individuals who experience a longstanding, internalized depression rooted in feelings of inadequacy and self-reproach. Such individuals often internalize relational conflicts and harbor an enduring sense of guilt, potentially stemming from early experiences of loss or deprivation rather than overt criticism from caregivers. Sara's idealization of work and family as "the centerpieces of my world" suggests a tendency to seek external validation.

Current Focus and Treatment Goals

At intake, Sara presented as a high-functioning professional grappling with the complex emotions surrounding her son's possible homosexuality, which she perceives as a threat to his salvation. Her primary concern is his spiritual welfare, as she fears he may jeopardize his relationship with God. She acknowledges a vague, persistent feeling of emotional "blah" but insists that her son's situation is her primary focus.

6 The Psychoanalytic Process

Building Rapport

Sara arrived precisely on time for her first session. Although the door to my office was open, she waited politely in the reception area until I came out to welcome her. Striking in appearance, with vivid blue eyes, all-white hair, and dressed professionally, Sara seemed to be in her mid-50s to early 60s. She greeted me with a warm smile and an upbeat demeanor, though her first words hinted at her unfamiliarity with the therapeutic process. "Okay, so I've never done this. What do we do?"

I explained that, like other relationships, our work would be rooted in trust, yet it would also remain professional – a safe, consistent space for her to share freely. Sara shared that she worked a lot and thought her anxiety and depression stemmed from concerns about her son, who might be gay. She was especially curious about my views on Biblical ethics and homosexuality. I responded thoughtfully, "When I talk to Christians, I don't always know where they're coming from. Saying 'Christian' is sort of like saying 'Asian food' – it establishes a category but doesn't tell me much specifically. I'd love to know more about your beliefs." Sara went on to share her deep faith and lifelong involvement in conservative Lutheran churches, a commitment her family had shared for generations. She confided, "I have no one to talk to." I sensed this was both a plea for understanding and an invitation to connect.

As Sara opened up, she recounted how she had discovered her son's diary and learned about his attraction toward men. She became tearful, confessing, "I'm worried he's going to lose his salvation. I think he's going to hell. This world is so brief, but eternity is forever." I took a moment to absorb the depth of her distress, setting aside any reflexive judgment to better empathize with her worldview. "This must

DOI: 10.4324/9781003653219-6

be unbearable for you," I said, acknowledging her pain. Encouraged, she shared more details. It felt as though I had passed a test, proving my willingness to listen without judgment.

Sara's distress had led her to her church's lead pastor, seeking reassurance. Instead, he reinforced her fears, suggesting that her son would likely go to hell and further ostracizing him by excluding him from communion. Devastated by the pastor's reaction, Sara had then turned to colleagues, who dismissed her concerns as overreaction and assured her that being gay was perfectly normal. In both instances, Sara felt invalidated and misunderstood, trapped between two polarizing views on her son's orientation. Our initial session became a crucial moment of connection, allowing her to feel seen and heard in a way that had been lacking.

Faith and Doubt

Taking this case to supervision, I was reminded that faith is not exclusive to religion but is a mental capacity, a notion that resonates in psychoanalytic thought. Reflecting on this in supervision, I realized that I had overlooked some foundational psychoanalytic concepts that could serve our work. Additionally, my supervisor advised that I would need to provide some psychoeducational support for Sara – a novel approach for me.

When I brought this back to Sara, we discussed the nature of faith as both a religious belief and a mental capacity, something that could grow and adapt. I shared a concept that I hoped would resonate with her: poet John Keats's "negative capability," which describes an ability to endure uncertainty and doubt without an immediate need for answers. Although this did not provide a direct solution, it opened a new dimension in our work. Together, we explored faith as a form of openness to life's unknowns – a way to remain present with pain and ambiguity rather than seeking quick answers.

Over time, our sessions deepened into a strong therapeutic alliance. As trust grew, Sara's curiosity led her to research me online, stumbling upon publicly accessible parts of my personal and professional profiles. She joked about "spying" on me, adding, "I saw your family pictures – you have a beautiful daughter." This glimpse into my life gave Sara a sense of connection, which she appreciated as someone deeply committed to family and parenting. She also remarked on my openness, reflecting that I wasn't afraid to be somewhat known, and it subtly fostered trust between us.

Goodness and the Black 'Blah'

As we continued, Sara shared experiences from her years as a nurse, describing the trials of emergency pediatric work and, more recently, her hospital's response during the COVID-19 pandemic. She spoke of the emotional toll of losing young patients, including a child who passed away without family present, a loss marked by a solemn ritual in which the staff lined the halls in silence. Hearing these stories, I was struck by Sara's courage and resilience. I began to recognize her enduring goodness and her deep commitment to care and service as key aspects of her identity.

Meanwhile, Sara's trust in me grew; I felt I had become a "third" space where she could be heard in a way that had been absent throughout her life. Our rapport allowed her to voice experiences that had previously been confined to unspoken realms.

One day, I asked about the source of her pain, inquiring if her suffering was solely related to her son. This led Sara to speak of an "internal black blah" – a formless, oppressive presence that she rarely articulated. Over subsequent sessions, she disclosed occasional suicidal thoughts, a source of guilt and shame. In response, we explored what it meant to consider suicide: was it an escape from the black blah, the pain, or perhaps a sense of contagion she feared would harm others? This dialogue opened a space to examine her suffering from multiple perspectives.

Sara bravely engaged with these questions, ultimately discerning that she wasn't seeking an end to herself but rather to aspects of her anguish. She began to describe specific emotions – sadness, anger, anxiety – uncovering distinct parts of what had once been an amorphous mass of pain. As we made the dark mass more digestible, piece by piece, it became less overwhelming. Underneath, a deeper fear surfaced: Sara worried she might be incapable of love.

This fear didn't align with my perception of her, as she appeared to genuinely love her family. But she admitted, "I don't know if I actually love them or if I'm just taking care of everyone so they don't feel the way I've felt all my life." It was a moment of profound self-reflection. Around this time, I received a rare text from Sara: "Thank you for all the work we're doing. I feel like I finally have someone to talk to. I wish I had a mini-you in my pocket growing up." In our next session, I thanked her for her kind words, but she politely declined to elaborate, indicating that she felt enough had already been said.

Toward a Transformed Sense of Self

As our work progressed, Sara's focus shifted from her son's potential homosexuality to her own emotional landscape, a transformation shaped by our mutual exploration of faith, her self-concept, and the underlying anxieties that had governed her life. Naming her emotions had enabled Sara to integrate aspects of herself, relieving the darkness that once loomed large. We ventured together into the depths of her inner world, and in the process, Sara gained a more nuanced understanding of her fears, her beliefs, and her capacity to love both herself and others.

Dream 1: Confrontation with the Shadow

Sara shared her first significant dream around this time. "There's a man," she began. "He's all black, like a shadowy ghost. In the dream, he's always there, no matter where I go or how fast I run. The faster I try to escape, the faster he catches up – even driving a car at one point. There's no way to escape him. I woke up terrified." I asked her about the emotions and associations she connected to this dream. Sara could name "fear" but couldn't offer much more. She had no clear associations to the figure.

I wondered if this could be a shadow aspect of our therapeutic work. Sara's reliance on our sessions was growing, and she seemed highly motivated by her need to care for others. Perhaps this dark figure represented an unnamed fear related to me or our work. Did she fear I might leave her? Or was it something deeper – a missing piece we hadn't yet addressed? I noted the dream, deciding to interpret it through a more Jungian lens, feeling a deep dive into a Kleinian interpretation might not resonate as effectively with her right now. Having recently emerged from a "black 'blah' space" internally, I sensed that an interpretation rooted in Jungian ideas could foster her curiosity without overwhelming her.

I explained to Sara that, after several months of analytic work, it's common for people to dream of shadow figures. In Jungian psychology, the early stages of analysis often involve facing one's shadow, which Jung (1981) describes as the unconscious parts of ourselves – those aspects lying outside the "light" of our ego. These shadow elements aren't necessarily negative; they're simply parts of us that we haven't named, explored, or understood yet (Jung, 2003). Sara was intrigued and began researching on her own. This period seemed to deepen our sessions, expanding our exploration of her internal world. Gradually, her internal black "blah" space found words and shape.

Together, we examined her shadow's personification – her perception of her own 'badness,' something she felt could almost "infect" others like a contagion. I wondered if this contagion fantasy stemmed from a hidden grandiosity: "I am so bad that my badness can affect others. I must protect them from it." Or, perhaps, it was a remnant of a paranoid-schizoid fantasy of omnipotence, along the lines of, "I control others' emotions." Both interpretations seemed to fit yet not quite. I considered Klein's work on primitive developmental states (Ogden, 1989) but decided against relaying these interpretations to Sara for now. Instead, I wanted to keep expanding our shared field of experience.

Drawing from cultural references, I pointed out how, in the Bible, an individual's ailment was often seen as more than personal – it could be linked to the well-being of a larger community, city, or even society. One person's sickness could reflect a collective malaise, connecting the personal to the communal. This expanded perspective seemed to lessen Sara's sense of burden, as we began exploring 'badness' not only in herself but in her environment. We talked about her 'badness,' Brent's 'badness,' the hospital's 'badness.' 'Badness' became an environmental condition rather than a sole defining trait.

From this conversation about 'badness,' our dialogue naturally evolved into one about 'goodness.' Just as shadow needs light, badness and goodness coexist in contrast. We discovered pairs of opposites forming in our sessions – goodness/badness, faith/doubt, shadow/light, homosexual/heterosexual, salvation/damnation, isolation/connection. These pairs weren't in opposition but could coexist, creating space for each other.

Through this exploration, Sara began to reflect that she wasn't all "bad" inside. She was able to experience and give love, something she had always done but hadn't been able to articulate or fully recognize. For the first time, she was able to put words to it and understand it more explicitly.

Dream 2: Loving, Living, Legacy

I asked Sara on several occasions if she was curious about where and when her shadow had emerged. By her account, her sense of 'badness' had always seemed to be an inherent part of her. She described her history as unremarkable, devoid of any clear trauma or loss that might explain this feeling. Sara acknowledged a compulsion to prioritize everyone else's needs above her own, a pattern that surely had origins somewhere. I chose not to press the matter and instead waited, allowing space for exploration. By this point, we had established a strong working alliance.

Together, we had developed a playful rapport, even creating a kind of "couple's language" that brought levity to our sessions. We often shared moments of laughter, especially while comparing anecdotes about raising toddlers. My feelings of warmth and respect for Sara continued to grow. I sensed her transference toward me was similarly warm, though perhaps tinged with an idealistic quality. While I cannot recall anything specific she said to support this impression, it was more of a subtle, intuitive feeling. Alongside this, I carried a quiet concern that she might, as she often did in other relationships – including her professional life – feel the need to take care of or please me. I kept an eye on this dynamic within our work together.

It was during this period that Sara shared her second dream. As an aside, I had often encouraged her to recall her dreams and to keep a dream journal, though she resisted these suggestions, and I chose not to push.

In recounting the dream, Sara said: "I am in the hospital being euthanized by my own choice. They've given me the injection, and I'm waiting for the poison to take effect. I'm wondering, 'What should I do with the time before I die? I think I should be doing something important, like writing a will, calling loved ones, or leaving something behind for someone else. But I have nothing to give.' The dream shifts. I am high above in a hot air balloon. Below me is a crowd. I don't know if it's a rock concert or a war. The dream shifts again. I am sitting on the couch with my parents. I am no longer in the hospital. I still have the opportunity to euthanize myself – I have the injection – but I don't use it. I think to myself, 'I need to find someone to love deeply, something worth really living and fighting for, and something of value to leave behind.'"

Sara described waking up and labeling this dream "The Three Ls: Loving, Living, and Legacy."

We spent many sessions exploring the meaning of this dream in relation to the other work we had been doing. Sara felt the euthanasia aspect reflected her suicidal thoughts, and I agreed. However, I also suggested that the dream might symbolize a larger internal shift – a *metanoia*, a transformative process often accompanied by images of death and renewal. I shared with her Hillman's (1998) *Suicide and the Soul*, which she found insightful.

I asked about her feelings and associations with the hot air balloon and the crowd below. She said she had no idea what these elements represented. I proposed that the hot air balloon might symbolize gaining a broader perspective, a bird's-eye view of her life. The crowd below could suggest a collective or social element, oscillating between creativity and celebration (the rock concert) and destruction and violence (the war). Sara resonated most strongly with the idea of the Three Ls.

She shared that she felt she hadn't been living her life fully. Though married, she did not feel she was loving fully. While she had material possessions to leave behind, she was unsure about what of deeper significance she could or should offer. Of the Three Ls, she was most uncertain about what she was living for.

I pointed out that, in the dream, the version of herself she encountered had the opportunity to end her life but ultimately chose not to. This, I suggested, was significant – a reflection of an inner choice to keep searching for meaning. Given the urgency of this theme, I encouraged her to elaborate further on it.

Balance and Bodyhood

For the first time, Sara recounted her numerous health conditions, both past and present. While she had mentioned a few of these in passing before, she had never discussed them in any sustained way. About seven years ago, she said, she simply collapsed at work. Fortunately, since she worked at a hospital, she was able to receive immediate medical attention. It took some time for the doctors to determine what was happening, but tests eventually revealed that she had lung cancer. While not immediately terminal, it was a type of cancer that would invariably return and, ultimately, become terminal. For now, Sara was stable, having undergone chemotherapy and multiple other treatments following her diagnosis.

More recently, she reported additional diagnoses: premature osteoporosis and a lump in her breast. Together, we used the time to explore what might be missing, what her body might be expressing or "bodying forth." Boss (1977) observed that we are always "bodying forth" our existences – an often-overlooked dimension in psychoanalysis. The role of our physical body, or "bodyhood," in both wellness and unwellness is too often neglected in a discipline that remains largely cerebral.

Sara and I had many discussions about her numerous health challenges, her present conditions, and her inevitable (as she described it) lung cancer recurrence. During this time, I suggested she read Mate's *When the Body Says No: Exploring the Stress-Disease Connection* (2011). Sara found the book particularly helpful. Mate described at length a personality type characterized by caregiving to the exclusion of self-care. This type of individual, Mate argued, experiences long-term stress that eventually manifests physically as cancer or other illnesses – a concept aligning with Boss's "bodying forth." Sara identified strongly with this caretaker archetype, and the book became a valuable adjunct to our work.

In time, our conversations shifted to focus on her work ethic. Sara had previously mentioned that she "worked a lot," but upon closer examination, it became clear that her work was literally nonstop. She managed two departments and had taken on an additional contract as the lead educator on COVID-19 for her region. She worked from sunrise, brought her work home in the evening, slept, and began again the next day. There was no work-life balance. Despite the immense good she had accomplished over decades, Sara felt that her work was killing her slowly.

I felt a protective instinct toward her, a desire to convince her to scale back. However, I restrained myself, placing faith in the process instead. During the peak of the pandemic, I focused on being there for her – supporting her as best I could. At times, I questioned whether this was "true" psychoanalytic work and brought it to supervision. My supervisor affirmed my approach, reminding me that, sometimes, analytic work involves being an encouraging, caring presence.

I wanted to help Sara reflect on her work ethic without judging her. After all, I was working a full-time job alongside my private practice. Though my schedule wasn't as extreme as hers, I recognized that I, too, was overworking. I would have been hypocritical to suggest she change without addressing my own habits.

Over time, I made a conscious effort to work less. Sara noticed this shift. While I didn't explicitly discuss it with her, she seemed to absorb what I was modeling. These changes coincided with a significant shift in her.

One day, she began a session by showing me pictures on her phone. "I'm thinking of starting a bed-and-breakfast. I might buy one of these houses," she said. I contained my surprise but expressed genuine interest in what had changed for her.

Sara admitted she wasn't entirely sure: "Something is just… [long silence] different." She explained that her husband was supportive of the idea and had always wanted to start a Christmas tree farm. Spontaneously, I said, "I can just see him driving around on his riding mower. Your sons are there, working on the farm. They don't have to work since they're working for you now." Sara laughed, picking up on the fantasy. This playful, imaginative space became an ongoing part of our work.

Without any direct prompting, Sara began to work less. She started going to work later and coming home earlier. She even kept a journal of the days she didn't bring work home and proudly shared it with me. The image that came to mind was of a plant beginning to sprout, breaking through the soil.

Interestingly, Sara never ended up purchasing a new house. Instead, her parents decided to downsize and offered to sell her their home and land for a nominal fee. They were waiting for their elderly horse to pass before moving, but the plan was set: Sara would start her bed-and-breakfast, and her husband would use the land for his Christmas tree farm.

It was during this transformative period that Sara brought another dream to our work.

Dream 3: Invisible Supports

> *Despite this invisible caring, we prefer to imagine ourselves thrown naked into the world, utterly vulnerable and fundamentally alone. It is easier to accept the story of heroic self-made development than the story that you may well be loved by this guiding providence, that you are needed for what you bring, and that you are sometimes fortuitously helped by it in situations of distress. May I state this as a bare and familiar fact without quoting a guru, witnessing for Christ, or claiming the miracle of recovery? Why not keep within psychology proper what once was called providence – being invisibly watched and watched over?*
>
> (Hillman, 1996 p. 39)

"I am driving to Linda's, having read her obituary online. I'm not sure how I came across it, but there I am. I arrive at Linda's house, go up to the front door, and walk in without knocking. Inside, there are men dressed in black suits. One of them approaches me, and I say, 'I'm not totally sure why I'm here, but I was a friend of Linda's.' The man replies, 'She had so many friends.' He smiles and says, 'Please, do what you need to here. Take your time.' I walk through the home, revisiting the many rooms and spaces where I spent so much time. I explore the garage, the yard, and everywhere else. Later, I come back into the house and see three men trying to move a grand piano. 'It's taking up too much space, and no one uses it anymore,' one of them says. 'Oh,' I reply, and then offer to help. They accept, and I help them lift and move the piano. Afterward, the dream shifts, and I find myself looking around the house again. This time, I am searching for something personal, something with Linda's handwriting. Finally, I find a small yellow Post-it note with her handwriting on it. I feel so happy, become tearful, and then wake up."

Sara grew tearful as she recounted the dream but had a subtle smile on her face. I sincerely thanked her for sharing it and asked her to provide some waking-life context to help me understand it better. Sara hesitated, then admitted there were aspects of her life she had kept private but now felt comfortable sharing. Before meeting her current husband, she had a significant relationship from ages 15 to 18, just prior to their relationship.

Sara revealed that she had never felt fully connected to her parents, particularly as an adolescent. "There was something missing at home," she confessed. I remarked that it was interesting how she had never spoken much about her upbringing, apart from describing it as outwardly "nice." Sara then explained how she fell in love with Gabrielle, Linda's son. "He gave me attention and somehow filled a void," she said. More than her feelings for Gabrielle, Sara explained that she had been drawn to his family, who had "adopted" her. She described their home as warm and welcoming, with Sunday dinners, extended relatives visiting, and a baby to play with. It was a source of belonging, love, and normalcy that she felt she lacked at home.

Without warning, Gabrielle ended their relationship. To this day, Sara doesn't know why. The family also cut off contact, and Sara said the loss of her "adoptive" family was more painful than the breakup itself. As she shared this, I felt a pang of sadness and told her I was deeply sorry she endured such a loss. I reflected that she must have been disconnected from her own feelings to miss signs of the impending separation.

Sara added that she had come across Linda's obituary two or three months ago while searching for information about the town where she and Gabrielle had dated. Seeing it was a shock. "I always thought I'd have time to speak to Linda again," she said. Sara admitted that she felt more connected to Linda than to Gabrielle, and she endorsed my observation that her relationship with Linda had held a deeper emotional resonance. Sara explained that she had kept this entire chapter of her life a secret, believing it better for her husband to think he was her only romantic partner. She also blamed herself for the breakup, despite no evidence to support this.

In the sessions that followed, we explored the dream together. I asked Sara about the house in the dream – what it looked like and how she felt seeing it again. Sara admitted that while she had never physically returned, she had looked it up online. She described her shock upon seeing it listed for sale, starkly empty compared to the vibrant home she remembered. "It was such a place of life," she said. Together, we explored the juxtaposition of "so much life" with the image of an "empty sold home."

While this contrast was difficult for Sara to bear, I pointed out the support she had received in the dream. The man in the dark suit welcomed her and encouraged her to take her time. Sara sat in thoughtful silence for a long moment before speaking. "You said earlier that my mind is on my side. I've never thought about it that way." I affirmed this and reflected that the dream seemed to provide her with support she hadn't recognized. "It's possible you're getting more support than you realize," I suggested. "Things may be better than they seem."

We turned our attention to the piano in the dream – heavy, unused, and taking up too much space. "You're letting go of things you don't need, making room for something new," I said. Sara engaged with this idea, identifying aspects of her life she wanted to release. I noticed her ability to reflect and differentiate her feelings was improving, as was her capacity for abstract and symbolic thinking.

During one session, I remarked that the third person helping move the piano might represent my supervisor, who had been instrumental in helping me navigate Sara's case. Sara was surprised. "I forgot you had a supervisor," she said. "It's strange to think I'm being supported even when I don't realize it." We discussed how, throughout her decades of nursing, she had spread goodness to countless people, both known and unknown. In turn, she had received support from unseen sources more often than she may have realized. This recognition seemed to deepen Sara's appreciation for the invisible supports in her life, both past and present.

Rupture and Repair

While things seemed to be going exceptionally well with Sara, changes were on the horizon. I had been successfully recruited to a position managing two methadone clinics in South Carolina. My wife and I had long been eager to leave Washington State for South Carolina, a location that felt more desirable for our family. At the time, I was working full-time at a local community mental health center while maintaining a small private practice. This new opportunity offered better pay and a chance for us to live where we truly wanted.

Despite my excitement, I was uncertain how Sara and my small group of patients would feel about the move. I discussed the situation in supervision, where my supervisor supported my decision. She emphasized the importance of taking care of my family and career while also noting that such a move could create ruptures in my analytic relationships.

When I broached the topic with Sara, we processed the decision together. I assured her that we could continue our sessions at the same frequency – three to four hours per week – via telehealth. Sara seemed reassured at first, but I couldn't shake the feeling that something was amiss.

After I moved, Sara soon expressed sadness about no longer meeting in person. She spoke of feeling let down and, at times, silly for feeling this way. I listened, saddened by the realization that I had hurt her feelings. I owned my part in her disappointment and expressed sincere regret. During this period, she also frequently asked about the possibility of me moving back to our other home in the Philippines. While my family had hopes of returning, the logistical challenges of traveling with a young child, compounded by restrictions at the time, made it impossible.

I found myself grappling with self-disappointment over the rupture I had caused. I brought the matter back to supervision, where my supervisor acknowledged the rupture but reassured me that such events are an inevitable part of the analytic process. She encouraged me to revisit Donald Winnicott's work, particularly in the context of rupture and repair.

I revisited Charles' (2017) *Introduction to Contemporary Psychoanalysis*, focusing on Winnicott's concepts. While familiar with Winnicott's work, revisiting it with fresh eyes proved invaluable. I began to see that, as much as I strive to avoid it, I may sometimes let my patients down. This is not to excuse such ruptures, but rather to highlight the importance of handling them thoughtfully.

My time in community mental health had accustomed me to a high turnover of patients and staff, a stark contrast to the depth and continuity required in psychoanalytic private practice. Winnicott's metaphor of the "good-enough mother" for analysis resonated deeply. I realized that regularity and stability were crucial for psychoanalytic patients and resolved to be more deliberate about providing those qualities moving forward.

In revisiting Winnicott's notions of holding, playing, and mutuality, I recognized another mistake I had made – I had been too focused on trying to alleviate Sara's disappointment. Instead, I decided to re-center our work on fostering her faith capacity. This shift created a new space for us to explore. Rather than dwelling on the rupture, I offered a holding space for Sara to process her feelings of loss and disappointment.

I was honored by Sara's willingness to share her disappointment so openly, and I told her so. This allowed me to sincerely apologize and take full responsibility for letting her down. Over time, Sara came to see me in a more realistic light, which neither of us had fully realized was necessary. Her idealizing transference became clearer through this process. While I had previously thought she had developed a healthy dependence, I came to see that I had underestimated the depth of her transference.

This experience taught me to be more mindful of such dynamics in the future. With time and effort, not only did Sara see me more realistically, but we also acknowledged that our relationship had grown stronger through the work of repairing the rupture. We found a new rhythm through telehealth, and since then, there have been no further significant ruptures.

Ultimately, this experience deepened my understanding of the therapeutic process, highlighting the value of repair in strengthening relationships and fostering growth – for both patient and therapist.

Survival Technique, Organizing Principle

It was sometime later that Sara brought up why she felt so disappointed. She explained that while there was nothing in her childhood she could recall as overtly traumatic or stressful, she had remembered something significant. Curious, I asked how she came to recall this memory. Sara explained that she often spent a great deal of time reflecting on our conversations between sessions. It was during one of these moments of reflection that her thoughts repeatedly returned to her father.

At first, she couldn't pinpoint why her mind wandered there – there were no specific images, memories, or even clear thoughts, just a general sense impression of her father. She described it as more of a feeling than anything else. She decided to sit with these impressions, and suddenly, a memory surfaced.

In this memory, Sara was about three years old, trying to get her father's attention. She described his response as what she called "polite attention," which she explained as offhand, vaguely positive acknowledgment, without any real engagement. As a father of a very gregarious toddler myself, I could empathize with such a response. While I tried to minimize it, I admitted that I, too, sometimes fell into that pattern: "Yes, honey. Uh-huh. That's great, sweetheart."

However, Sara clarified that this type of attention wasn't occasional for her father – it was the norm. I explained to her that genuine, focused parental attention serves as the "nutrients" a toddler's developing mind needs to thrive. As a nurse and someone passionate about parenting, Sara already understood this concept on some level, but she appreciated framing it in this way.

She seemed eager to share more about her memory. "I was able to get my dad's attention in a good way," she said. "Do you know how? I would do things to help him – like getting him things or fixing things, as much as a three-year-old could."

Here, a connection emerged: *If I help, I get the 'nutrients' I need.* This insight marked the emergence of what Sara and I came to recognize as a lifelong organizing principle. "You know," I pointed out, "toddlers think their parents are basically perfect. So, if something's wrong…" Sara finished my sentence: "…there was something wrong with me." The qualitative absence of her father's consistent, engaged presence had planted a belief in her that she was inherently flawed. To bypass this perceived flaw – at least in her childhood fantasy – she learned to earn her worth by helping others, especially her father.

Over time, this absence wasn't simply a quiet void; it expanded, growing in intensity as she aged. Alongside it grew an increasingly unconscious compulsion: to caretake, to enable, to perform acts of service for the greater good of others.

Eventually, Sara admitted, she could no longer discern whether her actions were motivated by a desire to protect others from her internal sense of black "blah" or by an attempt to earn small morsels of validation from those around her. Was she shielding others from her perceived contagious badness, or was she soliciting kindness through her relentless efforts to be a "good" woman – nurse, mother, wife, citizen?

"Maybe it's some combination of both," she said quietly.

The truth, she admitted, was that she could no longer tell.

Sara's Journey: Opening Up and Finding Rhythm

Sara was beginning to open up more, sharing experiences she had long kept buried. She recounted an attempted sexual assault by her uncle while they were alone on a trip together. Mercifully, she had been able to escape, but she had never spoken of the incident to anyone before now.

Sara also described a period during her battle with cancer when her husband had been emotionally distant. "It's not that he wasn't helpful," she said. "He was helpful. But he was so practical about it. 'Hey, let me know if you need help.' I thought that was just his way back then, but it really hurt not having any real support."

This perceived lack of support only reinforced Sara's belief in what she called her internal black "blah." She interpreted it as evidence of her inherent unworthiness. "After all," she said, "if I wasn't so bad, wouldn't he – or someone – have helped me or said something… anything?"

Once Sara recovered from cancer and her other physical ailments, the topic was never brought up again. "It was just sort of X-ed out, like it didn't happen," she said.

Sara's experiences with both her father and her husband left her with a sense that these pivotal relationships mirrored one another in their failures to provide consistent, supportive presence. This was particularly painful for Sara because, in her view, it also violated Biblical principles.

She referenced scripture, pointing out that the Bible commands husbands to demonstrate servant leadership:

Luke 22:24–26: Leading through service, not dominance.

Ephesians 5:23, 25–33: Loving one's wife as Christ loves the church.

Peter 3:7: Honoring one's wife and being understanding.

Sara understood these directives to mean that servant leadership includes, but is not limited to:

Serving one's family unconditionally.

Honoring the marriage covenant.

Resisting the urge to change one's spouse.

Prioritizing the family's needs over one's own.

Investing in personal growth and learning from others (Walker, 2016).

From both a psychoanalytic and Biblical perspective, Sara felt harmed. Psychologically, she struggled with the absence of emotional presence. Spiritually, she was confused and hurt by what she saw as a disregard for sacred principles.

As we continued processing her experiences, I introduced Sara to practical skills from Dialectical Behavior Therapy (DBT). These included strategies for setting boundaries, improving interpersonal effectiveness, and practicing healthy assertiveness.

The pace of our sessions slowed as Sara worked through the emotional weight of these memories. I saw no need to rush her. My supervisor offered insightful guidance about the natural ebb and flow of therapeutic progress, noting that it's common for patients to take a step back or slow down after delving into deeper material. This insight helped me stay attuned to Sara's process and honor the delicate balance between pressing forward and allowing space for reflection.

Thanks to the collaboration between supervision, Sara's perseverance, and my commitment to following her lead, we eventually found a rhythm that worked.

Voice and Vulnerability

The range of Sara's rhythm was expanding – our sessions were punctuated by more light-hearted laughter, deeper explorations, and a growing sense of calm familiarity. When we first met, the openness between us was understandably limited; we were strangers. Over time, however, our connection evolved into what could be described as *world-spanning openness* (DeRobertis, 2008), a sense of *thirdness* (Ben-Benjamin, 2007), the creation of an *intersubjective field* (Stolorow & Atwood, 1996), or even a kind of *mutual indwelling* (Schneider, 2007).

One day, after a session, I found myself reflecting on the process of working with Sara. An image of a wheel emerged in my mind. The wheel became a metaphor I could focus on and let evolve. In this image, Sara and I were the spokes, each extending from the wheel's center to its circumference. As the psychoanalytic work unfolded from session to session, the spokes generated a dynamic energy – a creative tension that connected the center and circumference.

This energy allowed the wheel to move, reflecting the nature of our work. Each session contributed to this motion by accumulating and releasing tension, a process essential for the wheel's character of movement. Without this mechanism – this collaboration between the spokes – there would be no mobility. The wheel would merely sit, inert and unused, waiting to be activated or discarded.

As I contemplated the wheel, another association surfaced: *perichoresis*, an ancient Greek term that translates roughly to "circle dance." In theological contexts, it describes the mutuality and relational flow within the Trinity. The word derives from *peri* (around) and *chorein*, which can mean "to make room for," "to go forward," or "to contain" (Ghosh, 2020).

This metaphor resonated deeply with me, and when I shared it with Sara, it sparked meaningful discussions. She was intrigued by the idea of *perichoresis*, and it became a fertile topic for exploration. The concept suggests a relational flow that has always existed – a mutuality of love and connection that predates creation itself. Within the Trinity, three persons share one substance, one flow, and one relationship. This eternal co-mutuality makes possible the human capacity to participate in that divine dance.

In many ways, the psychoanalytic process mirrors this "circle dance." Whether we call it *world-spanning openness, thirdness, intersubjective field, mutual indwelling*, my image of the hermeneutic wheel, or *perichoresis*, the relational dimension of psychoanalytic work is challenging to encapsulate. It is one of those experiences that must be felt to be understood – difficult to articulate without sounding, perhaps, a bit silly. Yet, in its ineffable way, it holds the essence of connection and transformation.

Processing Betrayal and Despair

As we discussed Sara's experiences, she revealed something deeply personal: not only did her husband remind her of her father and Gabrielle, but he had also had an affair. I gently asked if she would be comfortable sharing more. While Sara was recovering from lung cancer, her husband had an affair with a coworker. "It was about seven years ago, so I don't remember all the details," she said. "I think he confessed to it – I'm pretty sure he did. But I don't think I suspected anything before that. He blamed me. He said I was unattractive and that I forced him to have sex with someone else. Then he never mentioned it again."

I had many questions – about the length of the affair, whether it was his only one, or what might have led to it – but there were few answers. After his confession, Sara said the topic was dead. "He verbally assaulted me, and then it was just over," she explained. She never spoke of it again until this session. For Sara, it was yet another example of something critical in her life being, as she put it, "X-ed out."

In our ongoing work, we had been exploring relational dynamics and the mutual flow of connection, or *perichoresis*. But Sara's story also highlighted the impact of its absence, what might be called anti-*perichoresis* forces – the oppressive, isolating patterns that sever meaningful connection. The "primary background presence of identification," meant to nurture, had become tyrannical in her relationships.

Then Sara turned the focus to me: "And I let you down too when I moved."

I immediately understood how my relocation fit into her narrative of abandonment and betrayal – her father, Gabrielle, her husband. For the first time, Sara expressed anger. "Yes!" she yelled, and I was startled. I had never heard her raise her voice before. Her outburst caught me off guard, and I was admittedly apprehensive about the intensity of anger that had been buried alongside her internal black "blah." This "blah," which seemed to manifest physically in her cancer, now appeared to be surfacing as unrestrained fury. I feared what could happen if this energy turned outward – but at the same time, I hoped she would let it out, on her own terms.

I stayed composed – or at least appeared so. Sara's anger erupted in a torrent, a verbal geyser of emotions long repressed. Her face turned purple, her posture shifted as she leaned forward, half out of her chair, eyes bulging. I was momentarily concerned for her physical safety but felt that whatever was being expelled needed to run its course. The energy pouring from her, possibly into me through projective identification, felt charged with malice, hatred, and rage.

A line from Laing's *The Divided Self* (1965) surfaced in my mind: "Schizophrenia cannot be understood without understanding despair." In retrospect, I wondered if my unconscious had brought this to me for a reason, reminding me that despair is deeply tied to separateness, loneliness, and a longing to be understood.

I listened in silence as Sara's storm subsided. Those few moments felt like hours. I worried that the emotional purging could harm her, much like a fever or vomiting – necessary and potentially lifesaving, but capable of unintended damage if unchecked. Yet it felt like the right moment. Our relationship had enough containment to hold her in this vulnerable state.

As she sank back into her chair, quietly weeping, I leaned forward. Unlike her father, her uncle, Gabrielle, or her husband, I assured her that we were going to talk about it. Nothing she shared would be "X-ed out" of her experience. Here, everything was welcome in the circle dance of our work.

Note on Catharsis

It feels necessary to clarify that I am not suggesting Sara's intense emotional expression constituted a *classic* catharsis. Catharsis, as a concept, dates back to the early days of psychoanalysis, originating with Josef Breuer, who first developed it as a therapeutic goal. Breuer observed that when he hypnotized patients with hysteria, their degree of healing correlated with their ability to articulate past traumatic or otherwise unacceptable experiences. Breuer, a mentor and friend to Freud, co-authored *Studies on Hysteria* with him in 1895. This seminal work is widely considered the foundational text of psychoanalysis, and much of Freud's later career involved elaborating on the ideas imbued in him by Breuer.

In *Studies on Hysteria,* Freud and Breuer (2004) outline their theory and therapy for hysteria. They propose that hysterical symptoms often arise when an individual is exposed to a real or imagined trauma or other material deemed unacceptable to the conscious mind. To adapt, the psyche represses these contents – along with their associated affects. While this defensive maneuver protects the ego, it comes at the cost of suppressing the truth. This repression creates unconscious psychic conflict, which manifests as hysterical symptoms. In this model, catharsis is central to healing: it involves expelling the repressed psychic content and associated affects, thereby alleviating symptoms. Once the patient releases – or *cathects* – these contents, they can integrate the truth of their experience with less reliance on defensive strategies.

The case studies in *Studies on Hysteria,* such as that of Anna O., were groundbreaking for their time and held significant practical importance for the emerging field of nervous disorders. However, it could be argued that the landscape of psychopathology has shifted considerably since 1895, with certain conditions, such as the "glove complex," now virtually obsolete. Psychoanalysis has evolved through countless theories and developments, rendering the classical theory of catharsis more of historical interest than of contemporary practical utility.

That said, the broader ideas of psychic conflict, tension, and the need for release and reintegration remain relevant, especially in trauma work (Cieri & Esposito, 2019; Keiser, 2021; McGowan, 2014; Solms, 2018). Moreover, it is reasonable to assume that a psychoanalytic patient must often express previously inaccessible or unmanageable emotions as part of gaining conscious understanding. In Sara's case, her emotional outpouring seemed to emerge organically as part of a metanoia process – a fundamental shift in perspective and being – that should not be interrupted.

While classical catharsis is no longer a central focus in psychoanalysis, cathartic displays may still hold therapeutic value in the right context. Within the containment of a safe and consistent therapeutic frame, such expressions can facilitate healing and reintegration. Sara's experience, while not a textbook example of classic catharsis, was a form of catharsis – a release and reintegration of affect – within a larger process of working through her experiences.

Reorienting to the World

As Sara vented during our sessions, I found myself concerned about the potential risks of her emotions spiraling out of control. The mind, as Eigen (2021) observes, functions like a magnifying-minimizing machine, capable of amplifying or diminishing states. It's relatively easy to ignite such states, but exceedingly difficult – or even impossible – to halt them once in motion. Eigen writes:

> *Our minds are partly magnifying-minimizing machines. We use the term "to blow up" to characterize certain 'exaggerated' states. On the other side, I remember a patient who said she had a disappearing machine that made thoughts and feelings vanish… Our mind can maximize states and move towards zero at the same time, as well as develop maximizing-minimizing rhythms, a little akin to crescendo-decrescendo in music. Our mind can act like a plus-and-minus infinitizing machine blowing oneself up in both directions, intense and overflow and null. Maximum emotion and minimum emotion. Emotion moving towards infinity and emotion moving towards zero.* (p. 36)

Reflecting on Sara's emotional journey also brought to mind Heidegger's (2008) notion of orienting moments. Heidegger describes how humans typically live in a state of "they-self," absorbed in routines and the expectations of others. Occasionally, though, this they-self orientation is disrupted or shattered by profound experiences. In such moments, the individual is forcibly wrested from their they-self and everyday reality, thrust back upon themselves in a way that leaves them irrevocably transformed. This reorientation allows the person to return to their they-self, but with a more authentic and intentional engagement.

Heidegger also explores a related concept of encountering one's "ownmost self," describing it as a profound confrontation with the uncanniness of being. He writes:

> *In its who, the caller is definable by nothing "worldly." It is Dasein in its uncanniness, primordially thrown being-in-the-world, as not-*

> *at-home, the naked 'that' in the nothingness of the world. The caller is unfamiliar to the everyday they-self, it is something like an alien voice. What could be more alien to the they, lost in the manifold 'world' of its heedfulness, than the self individualized to itself in uncanniness thrown into nothingness? "It" calls, and yet gives the heedfully curious ears nothing to hear that could be passed along and publicly spoken about… The call does not report any facts; it calls without uttering anything. The call speaks in the uncanny mode of silence. And it does this only because in calling the one summoned, it does not call him into the public idle chatter of the they, but calls him back from that to the reticence of his existent potentiality-of-being. When the caller reaches him who is summoned, it does so with a cold assurance that is uncanny and by no means obvious.* (pp. 255–256)

While these moments can be disorienting and even dangerous, Sara's affective output fortunately remained contained within the safety of our relational frame. More importantly, she experienced an expansion of her emotional range – a realization that she could feel intense emotions and survive. Not only did she endure, but our therapeutic relationship also grew stronger as a result of the process. Sara demonstrated increasing affective and relational scope, evident in her occasional irritation and anger with me, which she expressed constructively. These were, in my view, clear signs of progress and wellness.

Sara began to consider whether she could express her rage toward her husband in a similar manner. Through our sessions, we explored her fantasies about confronting him. At times, she envisioned an explosive release – "I should just let him have it!" – while at other times, she leaned toward maintaining the status quo, recognizing the progress she had already made in therapy. Ultimately, we concluded that addressing the dynamics of her marriage would be best handled in the context of couples counseling. This decision felt right to both of us, as it preserved the focus of our work while providing another space to address her marital concerns.

In the meantime, we focused on interpersonal effectiveness, including boundary-setting, assertiveness training, and relational skills. Sara applied these techniques with her husband and at work, where she interacted with patients and colleagues. She was pleasantly surprised to find that most people, including her husband, responded positively to her newfound assertiveness and self-confidence.

Growth

Sara continued to demonstrate significant signs of improvement. As noted earlier, she experienced an *orienting moment* that allowed her to reorient herself toward her relationships and the world in a more authentic manner. This shift brought notable changes: she became more assertive, confident, maintained healthy boundaries, embraced spontaneity, and engaged with her affective life without being reactionary.

Sara's perception of me also evolved. I went from being the figure she wished she could have carried with her throughout childhood to someone she viewed through a more mature, differentiated lens. She was able to use our relationship as a platform to generalize dynamics, feelings, and relatedness to the broader world.

Interestingly, despite her presenting concern being her son's potential homosexuality, it became apparent that this was not an area Sara was organically drawn to explore in a sustained way. While I often took the initiative to bring up her son to honor her initial reason for seeking therapy, our focus naturally shifted to other matters. These issues, Sara discovered, were not random but followed a discernible pattern.

A Pattern of Functional Failures

Throughout her history, Sara identified multiple functional failures of primary background presences – her father, uncle, Gabrielle, me, and her husband. Initially, Sara described her childhood as idyllic and uneventful. However, over time, she revealed fragments of her experience that existed in a liminal space – truths she knew but didn't want to fully acknowledge. These revelations reflected an optimistic healing fiction Sara had clung to.

Supporting Sara's process required careful interpretation of her experiences and concerns in the immediacy of our sessions. I worked to ensure that my insights were accessible, requiring only one small step for Sara to understand and integrate them.

Through this work, Sara cultivated capacities for *faith, play,* and *acceptance.* For example, she became more comfortable with the uncertainty surrounding her son's sexuality, allowing it to simply *be* without tormenting herself with fears or assumptions. She learned to trust that something new could emerge in its own time. This ability to wait with faith extended into many areas of her life and relationships.

Discovering Play and Aloneness

Sara surprised me by taking photography classes – not casually, but by hiring an expert photographer for private lessons. She embraced the creative process, finding inspiration in her surroundings and sharing her images with others. Sara described moments of reverie while walking with her camera, which led us to discuss the capacity for being alone.

This concept, tied to primary background presences, resonated with Sara. Eigen (2011) notes:

> *As we grow, the aloneness that received nurturance supports us. A background aloneness, elusive and poignant, touches our beings. Part of what we do for each other, all through life, is to support the aloneness that informs and supports us.* (p. 93)

Similarly, Winnicott (1988) writes:

> *At the start is an essential aloneness. At the same time, this aloneness can only take place under maximum conditions of dependence… Throughout the life of an individual, there continues a fundamental, unalterable, and inherent aloneness.* (pp. 132–133)

We reflected on how Sara's early capacity for aloneness may have been disrupted. However, the focus was on her present ability to grow and enjoy this capacity. Beyond photography, Sara and her husband engaged in playful reverie about their future together, imagining their lives in the home they planned to acquire from her parents.

Improvements in Mental Health and Self-Understanding

Sara reported a complete absence of suicidal ideation, describing her depression as having "receded into the background." This shift reminded me of Eigen's (2005) concept of *psychic background radiation,* where the overwhelming force of past psychic explosions fades into a quieter, supportive presence.

Sara's increased focus on her physical health also reflected her newfound belief in her own importance. This was a striking shift from her earlier depressive worldview, characterized by thoughts like, "The world would be better off if I were dead." She had once compulsively performed good deeds in a desperate attempt to feel worthy.

Now, Sara understood her own agency and its value to herself and others. She committed to never letting anything be "X-ed" out again. Even if an experience was painful or confusing, she believed it could still be held, named, and given shape and understanding.

This transformation reflected Sara's growing resilience, authenticity, and capacity to live a fuller, more integrated life.

Termination

As of this writing, Sara and I continue working together, typically for four hours a week, never less than three. Recently, Sara has begun inquiring about reducing our session frequency. This feels appropriate, as she has made significant progress in her therapeutic journey. Currently, we are discussing the most thoughtful way to titrate her sessions, ensuring the process aligns with her background-attachment experiences. It is crucial that we approach this transition with sensitivity to her unique needs, though it seems timely for her to begin the process of separation. Sara is leading this shift, but I find myself curious about how her areas of growth intersect with her spiritual life.

One notable gap in our work is her relationship with God. While it is not essential that she share this aspect, I've noticed she seldom speaks about her faith or her walk with the Lord. This absence feels like a blank space in our therapeutic process and remains an area of curiosity for me. Additionally, I am intrigued by her dream life, which appears to hold rich, untapped material. However, Sara has been somewhat resistant to exploring this area further.

As previously mentioned, psychoanalytic faith functions as a clinical "sense organ," enabling the analyst to feel, see, and hear the patient's lived experience both during and between sessions. It also operates as a sensibility – a particular approach or attitude – toward the psychoanalytic process as a whole. This psychoanalytic phenomenological study has explored the sense and sensibility of faith within the treatment process.

Beginning with the foundational ideas of Bion and Eigen, the study incorporated insights from thinkers such as James Grotstein, Martin Heidegger, James Hillman, Carl Jung, and Thomas Ogden. Through a case study, it sought to elucidate the lived phenomena of psychoanalytic faith – both as sense and sensibility – within the therapeutic context. This hermeneutic case study, combined with the theoretical framework, provides a phenomenological "living picture" of how faith informs and shapes the psychoanalytic treatment process.

> *Faith plays an important role in transformational processes in psychotherapy. I don't mean "belief." Belief may be a necessary part of the human condition but it tends to prematurely organize processes that remain unknown. For me, faith supports experimental exploration, imaginative conjecture, experiential probes.* (Eigen, 2021, p. vii)

7 Psychoanalysis and the Sacred

On the Horizon of Contemporary Psychoanalysis

In the evolving world of psychoanalytic inquiry, existential-phenomenological psychoanalysis offers a compass for navigating human depth. Its future depends on our willingness to move beyond efficiency models and into spaces where slowness, presence, and depth are revalued. This modality will survive not through replication, but through care, reflection, and moral courage.

Clients do not present solely with symptoms; they present with histories, losses, and questions that resist formulation. Our task is not to name and tame experience but to dwell with it, to offer not judgment but presence. The future of this work is not scalability – it is sanctity of encounter.

Existential-phenomenological training must prioritize rigorous immersion in clinical philosophy. To read Heidegger or Binswanger clinically is not to cite them but to metabolize them. Philosophy is not a backdrop to analysis; it is part of its bloodline.

Faith in this framework is not an article of doctrine. It is the analyst's capacity to stay present when the patient has fallen silent or fallen apart. Faith is neither optimism nor persuasion; it is the quiet decision to remain in the room without needing to fix what is broken.

In the years to come, we will need analysts who are able to resist the pull of solutionism. We must stand as alternatives to automated therapeutics, standardized outcomes, and scripted engagements. The singularity of suffering demands the singularity of response.

Digital and pharmacological pressures will increase. Yet the soul's expression, its grief and longing, will not yield to medication or interface. There will remain a need for persons willing to attend to others in the dark – with neither light nor map, but with the steady flame of human presence.

DOI: 10.4324/9781003653219-7

Theological psychoanalysis will also rise as more seek integration between spirit and psyche. Here, concepts like grace, the unconscious, rupture, and healing meet not in tension, but in mutual deepening. We are not merely helping people cope. We are stewarding something sacred.

This is a future not of rapid progress but of ethical resistance. The analyst will remain one of the last figures in the helping professions who refuses distraction. We do not multitask healing. We pay attention – and in that attention, lives are altered.

Contemporary psychoanalysis must remain a place where people can confront suffering without being pathologized for it. Where questions can remain open. Where the analyst is not a mechanic but a midwife of truth. This future is worth building. And it begins again, each time we listen.

The Early Formation of Psychoanalysts: Training for Depth in an Age of Shallowness

The Analyst as Witness and the Sacredness of Encounter

As we move further into the future of contemporary psychoanalysis, one truth becomes increasingly clear: the role of the analyst is not reducible to that of clinician, technician, or interventionist. Rather, the analyst stands as a witness to the suffering of the other – a rare figure in an age marked by distraction and speed. This is not a passive role, nor a neutral one. To witness is to bear ethical responsibility; it is to hold space without exploitation, to remain attentive without intrusion, to recognize suffering without reducing it to symptomatology.

The future of psychoanalysis will belong to those who can safeguard this ethical commitment. In a cultural moment driven by metrics, efficiency, and consumer satisfaction, the analyst who resists these trends will do so not out of obstinance but out of care. We must preserve a place where suffering is not pathologized, where ambiguity is not something to be feared, and where human complexity is not flattened into diagnosis codes.

The sanctity of encounter remains the cornerstone of this future. Psychoanalysis, in its most fundamental expression, is an encounter between two subjectivities – an intersubjective space where transformation is made possible not by technique alone, but by presence, attention, and ethical regard. It is here that the analyst becomes something more than a professional. The analyst becomes a witness to the becoming of the other.

Psychoanalysis in the Age of Technological Reductionism

The cultural pressures facing psychoanalysis today are formidable. The rise of algorithmic therapeutics, artificial intelligence-driven mental health platforms, and pharmacological quick fixes have reshaped the landscape of care. These developments promise efficiency, scalability, and accessibility. Yet, they threaten to sever what is most essential in psychoanalytic work: the relational, the personal, the unpredictable.

In this emerging landscape, psychoanalysis risks being perceived as antiquated – too slow, too ambiguous, too human. And yet, it is precisely these qualities that render psychoanalysis indispensable. The work of analysis is inherently inefficient because human suffering is not reducible to input and output, to measurable data points, or to neatly resolved treatment plans.

The future of psychoanalysis depends on our refusal to be seduced by these technological promises. It will be sustained by those willing to advocate for slowness in an accelerating world, for ambiguity in an age of premature certainty, and for the irreducible singularity of human experience amidst the flattening tendencies of technological systems.

The Recovery of Philosophical Depth

If psychoanalysis is to endure, it must return to its philosophical roots. It is not enough to master technique or to memorize theoretical schools. Analysts must cultivate the capacity to think deeply and to engage rigorously with the philosophical traditions that inform their work. This requires an education that extends beyond the consulting room – one that draws from philosophy, theology, literature, and the broader human sciences.

The analyst of the future must be conversant not only in the language of symptoms but in the language of existence. They must be able to read Heidegger and Binswanger, Merleau-Ponty and Laing, not as distant theorists but as fellow travelers in the project of understanding human being. Philosophy is not a luxury in this regard; it is a necessity. Without it, psychoanalysis risks becoming hollow – a collection of techniques without depth, interventions without understanding.

Psychoanalysis is, at its heart, a philosophy of human life, of human suffering, and of human possibility. To forget this is to forget the ethical and existential stakes of the analytic task.

The future of psychoanalysis depends upon the formation of analysts who are willing and able to do this kind of work. This requires a training process that is as much ethical and existential as it is technical and theoretical. Analysts must undergo their own analysis not merely as a requirement for certification but as a crucible for their own becoming. They must learn to confront their own defenses, their own histories of suffering and survival, in order to become capable of bearing the suffering of others.

Training must also include a deep engagement with philosophy, literature, and theology. Analysts cannot afford to be merely clinicians; they must be thinkers, readers, and persons of ethical depth. They must cultivate the capacity to think deeply about the human condition, to engage rigorously with the questions that animate human life, and to tolerate the ambiguity that inevitably accompanies those questions.

In an age that prizes speed, efficiency, and certainty, the training of analysts must resist these cultural pressures. It must be a slow, demanding process that shapes not only the analyst's knowledge but their character. Only in this way can psychoanalysis remain a place where the complexity and mystery of human life are honored and engaged.

In the early days of psychoanalysis, long before the discipline was shaped by regulatory boards, standardized curricula, and professional associations, the formation of an analyst was understood to be an ethical, intellectual, and existential undertaking. It was not simply a matter of learning technique; it was a process of becoming – of submitting oneself to the slow, often painful work of self-examination, philosophical reflection, and ethical deepening.

Analysts were not trained in the modern, institutional sense. There were no certification exams, no accreditation bodies, no rigid protocols. Instead, psychoanalytic formation unfolded through relationships, mentorships, and, most importantly, through personal analysis. The first analysts – Freud, Jung, Ferenczi, Abraham, and their early colleagues – learned the craft of analysis not in classrooms but in salons, correspondence, and intimate conversations. They read deeply, argued passionately, and engaged in sustained dialogue about the nature of human suffering and transformation.

Personal analysis was not a bureaucratic checkbox; it was the cornerstone of training. It was understood that one could not sit with the suffering of others without first confronting one's own unconscious life. The analytic process was arduous, unpredictable, and profoundly personal. It shaped the analyst not merely as a clinician but as a human being capable of bearing witness to the fragility and complexity of others.

Equally essential was the intellectual breadth expected of early analysts. They were readers of philosophy, literature, mythology, and religion. Freud drew from Greek tragedy and Enlightenment rationalism; Jung immersed himself in alchemy and the mystic traditions; Binswanger and Boss read Heidegger. Analysts were expected to engage with the great questions of existence – not only what causes symptoms but what it means to live, to love, to suffer, and to die. Psychoanalysis was never merely a method; it was a way of engaging the mystery of human being.

Training in those early decades was rooted in apprenticeship, philosophical reflection, and ethical formation. The analyst was understood to be a witness, a companion, a fellow traveler – not an expert delivering diagnoses or treatments. Knowledge was passed not through formal instruction but through dialogue, personal analysis, and the shared labor of confronting the unconscious.

This early ethos has largely been lost. As psychoanalysis became professionalized in the mid-twentieth century, it was folded into psychiatric institutions, standardized training programs, and bureaucratic credentialing systems. What was once a practice of ethical formation and philosophical reflection became, in many places, a technique to be mastered, a credential to be obtained.

But the heart of psychoanalysis remains in those early commitments: to slowness, to depth, to ethical presence, to the irreducibility of human life. The future of psychoanalysis will depend on our willingness to recover these roots – to form analysts not only as technicians but as thinkers, listeners, and witnesses to the human soul.

Reawakening Mystery in Contemporary Psychoanalysis

The growing emergence of contemporary psychoanalysis is not incidental. It reflects a broader cultural need to reclaim dimensions of human experience that have been neglected in the secular, clinical models of care. This is not a call to impose belief systems upon the analytic encounter. Rather, it is an invitation to recognize that beneath the suffering of the analysand often lies a deeper longing – a longing for meaning, for belonging, for connection with something greater.

Contemporary psychoanalysis does not resolve this longing; it makes space for it. It acknowledges that human suffering is not merely psychological but existential, that the human condition is marked by a tension between finitude and transcendence. In this way, contemporary psychoanalysis offers a corrective to the reductionism of contemporary clinical discourse. It invites analysts to engage with mystery, to approach the human soul with reverence, and to hold space for questions that have no easy answers.

On Ethical Resistance and the Analyst's Responsibility

The future of psychoanalysis will not be secured through institutional authority or technological innovation. It will be safeguarded by analysts who embody ethical resistance – who refuse to collude with systems that commodify suffering, who resist the urge to diagnose away complexity, and who remain steadfast in their commitment to human presence.

This resistance is not loud or dramatic. It is the quiet refusal to abandon the singularity of the other. It is the decision to pay attention when distraction would be easier, to remain curious when certainty tempts, and to bear witness when silence becomes heavy.

The analyst's responsibility, in this sense, is not merely clinical; it is moral. It is the responsibility to create and preserve spaces where human suffering can be spoken without fear, where ambiguity is permitted, and where healing is understood not as the elimination of pain but as the possibility of renewed presence.

A Future Worth Building

In the end, the future of contemporary psychoanalysis will be shaped not by its capacity to conform to the demands of the market or the metrics of efficiency, but by its capacity to remain faithful to its deepest commitments. This is a future that will not be measured in profits or productivity but in lives quietly altered through the patient work of attention and care.

It is a future that values slowness over speed, depth over immediacy, relationship over technique. It is a future in which the analyst stands not as an expert or authority but as a fellow traveler – one willing to listen, to stay, and to bear witness.

This future is worth building. It is worth defending. And it begins again, each time an analyst chooses to pay attention, to hold space, and to honor the mystery and dignity of the human soul.

In the evolving landscape of contemporary psychoanalysis, the question of meaning cannot be ignored. The analytic space has always been more than a place to relieve symptoms or interpret dreams; it has been a place where meaning itself is formed, questioned, lost, and reconstituted. As the future of psychoanalysis unfolds, analysts must return to this fundamental truth: analysis is a meaning-making, meaning-discovering endeavor. It is not a clinical intervention in the reductive sense, but an ethical encounter with the suffering other. What distinguishes psychoanalysis from adjacent forms of care is its willingness to remain with the patient in the space of not-knowing, in the ambiguity of longing and loss. It is here, in the refusal to impose resolution, that meaning begins to emerge – not as something given, but as something discovered, co-created in the analytic field. This requires of the analyst a particular kind of presence. It is not enough to understand the structures of the psyche or to master the tools of interpretation. The analyst must cultivate the capacity to remain open, to resist the pull of premature closure, and to bear witness to the patient's struggle without defense. This is an ethical vocation, one that demands courage, patience, and deep humility. In a cultural moment dominated by the logics of efficiency, measurement, and technological mediation, the psychoanalytic encounter remains one of the few places where the irreducible singularity of human suffering is honored. It is a sacred space, not in a religious sense, but in the sense that it protects something fragile and essential: the mystery of the human soul.

Psychoanalysis and the Recovery of Human Being-in-the-World

The future of psychoanalysis will be determined by its capacity to defend and reclaim something that has become increasingly endangered in modern life: the presence of one person fully with another. In a world awash in technological distraction, instantaneous communication, and algorithmic prediction, the ability to offer sustained, undivided attention has become rare. Yet, it is precisely this form of presence that is the foundation of the psychoanalytic encounter.

Psychoanalysis is, at its heart, a discipline of listening – not listening merely for content or symptom but for the subtle rhythms of another person's being. It is a listening that requires patience, attunement, and the capacity to tolerate uncertainty. It is a listening that refuses to interrupt, correct, or explain prematurely. In the consulting room, this form of attention is not an incidental courtesy; it is the primary means by which healing becomes possible.

In the years ahead, as mental health care becomes increasingly mechanized and standardized, analysts will be called to defend this simple, radical act: to remain present, to listen deeply, and to refuse the reduction of the human subject to a set of clinical data points. This is not an act of nostalgia but an ethical imperative. The analyst who listens in this way resists the forces that commodify suffering and deny the irreducible complexity of human life.

The Analyst as Ethical Witness

To occupy the analytic position is not merely to apply a set of technical skills; it is to assume a particular ethical posture. The analyst is not a mechanic, technician, or even an expert in the traditional sense. The analyst is a witness – one who stands alongside the patient without the need to control, interpret, or solve.

This ethical stance requires the analyst to surrender the fantasy of mastery. It requires a willingness to remain in the presence of suffering without defense, without evasion, without recourse to premature explanation. It is an act of faith to listen in this way, to allow the patient's story to unfold in its own time, according to its own rhythms.

In the analytic encounter, the analyst bears witness not only to the patient's suffering but also to their becoming. The analyst listens for what is not yet spoken, for the faint stirrings of transformation that emerge in the silence between words. This is sacred work – not in a theological sense, but in the sense that it honors the dignity and singularity of the human soul.

Toward a Deepening Ethic of Care in Contemporary Psychoanalysis

The integration of philosophical and theological reflection into psychoanalytic practice represents one of the most promising avenues for the future of depth work. Contemporary psychoanalysis' sense of faith does not seek to impose religious belief upon the analytic situation. Rather, it acknowledges that the questions patients bring to analysis – questions of suffering, meaning, love, loss, and transformation – are often theological in nature, even when they are not framed in explicitly religious terms.

By attending to the spiritual dimensions of human experience, contemporary psychoanalysis expands the scope of analytic care. It invites the analyst to engage with the patient's longing for transcendence, belonging, and grace. It makes space for the recognition that beneath clinical symptoms often lies a deeper spiritual hunger.

This approach does not require the analyst to become a theologian or spiritual guide. It requires only the willingness to hold open the possibility that the analytic encounter touches upon something larger than the individual psyche – that in the work of analysis, something sacred is at stake.

As psychoanalysis moves deeper into the twenty-first century, it becomes clear that its survival and relevance will not depend upon how well it conforms to prevailing cultural demands but rather upon how courageously it resists them. This discipline was never meant to align with the logics of productivity, efficiency, or commodification. It has always been, at its heart, a radical, patient, and deeply human endeavor. In an era where the human is increasingly displaced by data, where the soul is reduced to metrics, psychoanalysis stands as one of the last spaces where people may bring the whole of their being – fractured, longing, unfinished – without fear of reduction.

What psychoanalysis offers is something more enduring than symptom relief. It offers the possibility of bearing witness to one's own life in the company of another. It invites individuals to tell the story that cannot be told anywhere else, to articulate what has remained unspeakable, to confront what has been disavowed. This is not a mechanical task but an ethical and existential undertaking.

In the years to come, it will become increasingly clear that the analyst's task is not simply to intervene, interpret, or correct. It is to dwell alongside the analysand in the dark and unlit corners of their life, to make space for ambiguity, sorrow, contradiction, and longing. In doing so, the analyst affirms something that cannot be measured or monetized: the dignity and irreducibility of the human soul.

The future of psychoanalysis is not assured. It will survive only if those who practice and teach it are willing to preserve its ethical core. This will require moral courage – a refusal to submit to the flattening forces of the marketplace, the insurance industry, and algorithmic therapeutics. It will require the cultivation of a new generation of analysts who understand that their primary task is not to provide solutions but to offer presence.

The work is slow. It is often thankless. It requires stamina, curiosity, and deep humility. And yet, it is in this slowness that something essential is preserved – a space where human suffering can be spoken without fear, where the analyst remains attentive not to outcomes but to the singular unfolding of another person's life. In a world of noise, this quiet work is revolutionary.

If psychoanalysis is to endure, it must reclaim its rightful place as an ethical, philosophical, and spiritual practice – not merely a clinical technique but a way of being with others that honors the complexity and mystery of human existence. The analyst's office, increasingly, will be one of the few places where individuals are not asked to justify their suffering, not required to package their experiences into digestible soundbites, but are instead invited to linger in the ambiguity of their own becoming.

Beyond the Couch: Evolving Psychoanalytic Horizons

The next generation of psychoanalysts must be trained not only in theory and technique but in the formation of their very being. They must learn to listen beyond words, to recognize the texture and timbre of suffering without defensiveness or the need for premature resolution. This requires more than intellectual mastery; it requires existential depth.

Contemporary psychoanalysis will have a vital role to play in this future. As the fragmentation of meaning accelerates in the broader culture, many will turn again to questions of spirit, grace, and the unconscious yearning for something beyond mere survival. Psychoanalysis, when practiced thoughtfully, can meet this longing – not with doctrine, but with the capacity to hold space for the sacred dimensions of human life.

Such work will not be easy. It will require analysts who are willing to enter into the depths of human despair without pretense, to bear witness to the pain of the other without resorting to diagnosis or solutionism. It will require training programs that emphasize ethical formation, philosophical reflection, and the analyst's own ongoing analysis.

But the rewards of such labor cannot be overstated. In a culture increasingly marked by alienation, loneliness, and superficiality, psychoanalysis offers something rare: a relationship in which one's suffering is not pathologized but taken seriously; in which one's questions are not answered prematurely but are allowed to unfold; in which one's existence is affirmed not through productivity but through presence.

This is the vocation of psychoanalysis – not to fix but to listen, not to resolve but to accompany. It is a vocation rooted in the radical belief that to pay attention to another person's suffering, without judgment or agenda, is itself a form of healing.

The future of psychoanalysis will depend on our ability to remain faithful to this vocation. It will require us to resist the cultural forces that would render human beings into data points, to create spaces where suffering can be spoken without fear, and to cultivate the ethical and philosophical depth necessary to meet the complexity of human life.

At the center of psychoanalysis lies an irreducible paradox: the analyst is charged with facilitating transformation without imposing it, with listening deeply while withholding judgment, with holding the suffering of the other without collapsing into rescue. This paradox is not an obstacle to the analytic process; it is its very ground. It is within this tension that psychoanalysis reveals itself not as a science of the mind, but as an ethical and philosophical practice concerned with what it means to be human.

The analyst's responsibility, then, is not to deliver answers but to remain in the presence of questions. This requires an extraordinary capacity for restraint – a refusal to interrupt, to categorize, to simplify. It requires a deep attunement to the ways in which suffering often resists articulation, how it reveals itself only slowly, in fragments, in the gaps between words.

The cultural forces arrayed against this practice are formidable. Everywhere, there is a demand for certainty, for speed, for efficiency. Mental health care increasingly bends toward the logic of productivity, offering quick solutions, diagnostic clarity, and measurable outcomes. In such an environment, psychoanalysis can appear obsolete, too slow, too ambiguous, too human.

Yet it is precisely these qualities that render psychoanalysis indispensable. The analytic space is one of the last remaining places where ambiguity is permitted, where complexity is not feared, where suffering is not commodified. It is a space where individuals can encounter themselves – not as problems to be solved but as beings in process, in flux, in search.

For this reason, the training of future analysts must prioritize not only theoretical knowledge but the cultivation of ethical sensibilities. Analysts must be shaped by their own encounters with suffering, by their own analysis, by sustained philosophical reflection. They must be prepared not only to interpret but to listen, not only to analyze but to accompany.

Contemporary psychoanalysis offers one powerful way forward. By integrating the ethical and spiritual dimensions of human life, it reclaims psychoanalysis as a practice concerned with the whole person – not just the psyche, but the soul. It invites analysts to recognize that beneath the patient's symptoms often lies a deeper longing: a longing for grace, for belonging, for the possibility of being seen and known.

This approach does not require analysts to become theologians or spiritual guides. It requires only that they remain open to the sacred dimensions of human experience, that they recognize the ways in which suffering often gestures toward something beyond itself. In doing so, they restore psychoanalysis to its rightful place – not as a technique or intervention but as a vocation rooted in presence, patience, and care.

One of the quiet dangers that psychoanalysis will continue to face in the years ahead is its potential co-optation by institutional systems that seek to tame its radical core. Managed care, regulatory bodies, and academic credentialing institutions often demand that psychoanalysis conform to their preferred models of accountability and standardization. But psychoanalysis, by its very nature, resists such containment. It is not an intervention to be measured or a procedure to be streamlined. It is an ethical practice of presence – a practice that refuses to treat suffering as something to be controlled.

The analyst's task, therefore, is to guard against the slow erosion of the discipline's ethical and philosophical commitments. This is not simply a matter of preserving an intellectual tradition; it is a matter of safeguarding the conditions under which genuine healing can occur. Analysts must remain vigilant against the pressures to professionalize, commodify, or bureaucratize the analytic encounter.

This vigilance is not merely defensive. It is creative. It requires analysts to reimagine what psychoanalysis can be in the contemporary world. It requires them to forge new ways of practicing, teaching, and writing that remain faithful to the discipline's ethical heart while responding to the realities of the present moment.

One promising avenue for this reimagining is the continued development of contemporary psychoanalysis. By drawing upon the rich resources of spiritual and philosophical traditions, analysts can deepen their understanding of human suffering and renewal. They can create spaces in which questions of meaning, belonging, and grace are not pathologized but welcomed.

In these spaces, the analyst does not offer answers. They offer presence. They offer the possibility of a relationship in which suffering can be spoken, heard, and held without being resolved. They offer a place where the analysand can confront not only their symptoms but their existence – their longings, their fears, their search for a life worth living.

This is a practice that requires more than technical competence. It requires ethical and existential maturity. It requires the analyst to undergo their own process of becoming, to engage with their own suffering and questions, to cultivate the humility and patience necessary to accompany others on their journeys.

In a world increasingly driven by speed, efficiency, and distraction, psychoanalysis offers something precious: slowness, attention, care. It invites us to dwell with what is difficult, to remain present to what is painful, to honor the mystery and complexity of human life. This is not a luxury. It is an ethical necessity.

The future of psychoanalysis will belong to those who can hold this space – to those who refuse to trade presence for productivity, ambiguity for certainty, care for efficiency. It will belong to those who recognize that in listening deeply to another person's suffering, something sacred is preserved.

As we consider the trajectory of psychoanalysis in the decades to come, one essential truth emerges: the future of this practice will not be secured through institutional expansion, technological integration, or professional recognition alone. It will be secured through the quality of the encounter between analyst and analysand – through the capacity of analysts to remain steadfast in their commitment to human depth, ethical presence, and the irreducibility of suffering.

This is a future that demands more than theoretical sophistication. It demands analysts who are willing to risk their own comfort, to relinquish the illusion of mastery, to enter fully into the lived realities of those who come seeking help. It demands analysts who can tolerate the discomfort of ambiguity, who can remain present in the face of suffering without defense or distraction.

The cultivation of such analysts will require a reorientation of training and education. Rather than focusing solely on technical skill acquisition or theoretical memorization, analytic training must foreground the ethical, philosophical, and spiritual dimensions of the work. Candidates must be encouraged not only to learn but to become – to undergo their own analytic journeys, to confront their own histories, to grapple with the questions that animate human existence.

In this context, the integration of contemporary psychoanalysis will be vital. As the cultural fragmentation of meaning continues to accelerate, patients will increasingly bring into the analytic space not only their psychological wounds but also their existential longings. They will bring questions of belonging, grace, rupture, and renewal – questions that cannot be answered by clinical technique alone.

The analyst who is prepared to meet these questions will not do so with doctrine or dogma but with presence and humility. They will understand that healing does not reside in explanation but in encounter. They will recognize that the analytic space is one of the few remaining places where the human soul can be taken seriously – where suffering is neither pathologized nor dismissed but engaged with care and reverence.

This is a demanding future. It requires analysts who are willing to dwell in uncertainty, who are able to accompany others without imposing their own agendas, who are attuned to the ethical stakes of their work. But it is also a hopeful future. For in this work, something essential is preserved: the dignity of human suffering, the possibility of transformation, the affirmation of presence over product.

Psychoanalysis will not survive because it has adapted to the demands of the marketplace or the metrics of efficiency. It will survive because there remain those who believe in the value of deep listening, of ethical presence, of human care. It will survive because there remain those who are willing to do the slow, difficult, and essential work of being with others in their suffering.

And in that work, psychoanalysis will continue to bear witness to the enduring mystery of what it means to be a human being.

In the end, faith is not what we believed it would be. It is not the clarity we once begged for, nor the certitude we once envied in others. It is not the pristine logic of systems, nor the emotional anesthesia of creeds. Faith, rather, is what remains when every system has cracked, every defense has thinned, and we are left again with that quiet, stubborn impulse to trust something we cannot name.

Theological psychoanalysis has taught us that the psyche does not move in straight lines. Neither does the soul. The sacred is not found by climbing upward, but often by descending – into the body, the wound, the silence. We do not transcend our humanity to find faith. We become more human. We listen to our dreams. We forgive our brokenness. We re-enter the shattered narratives, this time without flinching.

Faith is not the absence of doubt. It is what gives us the courage to bear doubt without collapsing. It is the relational field that allows us to speak even when our voice trembles. It is the presence that holds us when the words fail. And when no one is watching – when we are alone with our unknowing – it is the faint warmth that does not leave.

The journey mapped in these pages is not one of conquest but of return. Not the return to answers, but to presence. To lived experience. To that strange, sacred unfolding of the self in the presence of something more. We may call it God. We may not. But we have stood near its edges. We have breathed in its absence. We have wept in its nearness.

Psychoanalysis listens for what theology has sometimes missed: the sound of the soul, unspeakable, irreducible, raw. But theology listens too – for the cry, the whisper, the presence that calls us even in the dark. Together, they ask not that we solve the mystery of existence, but that we dwell within it. And to dwell is not to fix – it is to remain. To risk love. To risk meaning. To risk being.

Faith, in the end, is not a conclusion but a continual beginning. A posture of openness. A stance of return. A willingness to be wounded by beauty. It is the courage to walk through a life that does not explain itself – and to listen anyway. It is, as Michael Eigen says, "a contact with life itself." No more, no less.

May your faith live not in what you have captured, but in what you have released. Not in your certainties, but in your surrender. Not in the perfection of your beliefs, but in the aliveness of your being.

8 Holding the Tension of the Opposites, Making Room

Beyond the Couch: Evolving Psychoanalytic Horizons

The next generation of psychoanalysts must be trained not only in theory and technique but in the formation of their very being. They must learn to listen beyond words, to recognize the texture and timbre of suffering without defensiveness or the need for premature resolution. This requires more than intellectual mastery; it requires existential depth.

Contemporary psychoanalysis will have a vital role to play in this future. As the fragmentation of meaning accelerates in the broader culture, many will turn again to questions of spirit, grace, and the unconscious yearning for something beyond mere survival. Psychoanalysis, when practiced thoughtfully, can meet this longing – not with doctrine, but with the capacity to hold space for the sacred dimensions of human life.

Such work will not be easy. It will require analysts who are willing to enter into the depths of human despair without pretense, to bear witness to the pain of the other without resorting to diagnosis or solutionism. It will require training programs that emphasize ethical formation, philosophical reflection, and the analyst's own ongoing analysis.

But the rewards of such labor cannot be overstated. In a culture increasingly marked by alienation, loneliness, and superficiality, psychoanalysis offers something rare: a relationship in which one's suffering is not pathologized but taken seriously; in which one's questions are not answered prematurely but are allowed to unfold; in which one's existence is affirmed not through productivity but through presence.

This is the vocation of psychoanalysis – not to fix but to listen, not to resolve but to accompany. It is a vocation rooted in the radical

DOI: 10.4324/9781003653219-8

belief that to pay attention to another person's suffering, without judgment or agenda, is itself a form of healing.

The future of psychoanalysis will depend on our ability to remain faithful to this vocation. It will require us to resist the cultural forces that would render human beings into data points, to create spaces where suffering can be spoken without fear, and to cultivate the ethical and philosophical depth necessary to meet the complexity of human life.

At the center of psychoanalysis lies an irreducible paradox: the analyst is charged with facilitating transformation without imposing it, with listening deeply while withholding judgment, with holding the suffering of the other without collapsing into rescue. This paradox is not an obstacle to the analytic process; it is its very ground. It is within this tension that psychoanalysis reveals itself not as a science of the mind, but as an ethical and philosophical practice concerned with what it means to be human.

The analyst's responsibility, then, is not to deliver answers but to remain in the presence of questions. This requires an extraordinary capacity for restraint – a refusal to interrupt, to categorize, to simplify. It requires a deep attunement to the ways in which suffering often resists articulation, how it reveals itself only slowly, in fragments, in the gaps between words.

The cultural forces arrayed against this practice are formidable. Everywhere, there is a demand for certainty, for speed, for efficiency. Mental health care increasingly bends toward the logic of productivity, offering quick solutions, diagnostic clarity, and measurable outcomes. In such an environment, psychoanalysis can appear obsolete, too slow, too ambiguous, too human.

Yet it is precisely these qualities that render psychoanalysis indispensable. The analytic space is one of the last remaining places where ambiguity is permitted, where complexity is not feared, where suffering is not commodified. It is a space where individuals can encounter themselves – not as problems to be solved but as beings in process, in flux, in search.

For this reason, the training of future analysts must prioritize not only theoretical knowledge but the cultivation of ethical sensibilities. Analysts must be shaped by their own encounters with suffering, by their own analysis, by sustained philosophical reflection. They must be prepared not only to interpret but to listen, not only to analyze but to accompany.

Contemporary psychoanalysis offers one powerful way forward. By integrating the ethical and spiritual dimensions of human life, it reclaims psychoanalysis as a practice concerned with the whole person – not just the psyche, but the soul. It invites analysts to recognize that beneath the patient's symptoms often lies a deeper longing: a longing for grace, for belonging, for the possibility of being seen and known.

This approach does not require analysts to become theologians or spiritual guides. It requires only that they remain open to the sacred dimensions of human experience, that they recognize the ways in which suffering often gestures toward something beyond itself. In doing so, they restore psychoanalysis to its rightful place – not as a technique or intervention but as a vocation rooted in presence, patience, and care.

One of the quiet dangers that psychoanalysis will continue to face in the years ahead is its potential co-optation by institutional systems that seek to tame its radical core. Managed care, regulatory bodies, and academic credentialing institutions often demand that psychoanalysis conform to their preferred models of accountability and standardization. But psychoanalysis, by its very nature, resists such containment. It is not an intervention to be measured or a procedure to be streamlined. It is an ethical practice of presence – a practice that refuses to treat suffering as something to be controlled.

The analyst's task, therefore, is to guard against the slow erosion of the discipline's ethical and philosophical commitments. This is not simply a matter of preserving an intellectual tradition; it is a matter of safeguarding the conditions under which genuine healing can occur. Analysts must remain vigilant against the pressures to professionalize, commodify, or bureaucratize the analytic encounter.

This vigilance is not merely defensive. It is creative. It requires analysts to reimagine what psychoanalysis can be in the contemporary world. It requires them to forge new ways of practicing, teaching, and writing that remain faithful to the discipline's ethical heart while responding to the realities of the present moment.

One promising avenue for this reimagining is the continued development of contemporary psychoanalysis. By drawing upon the rich resources of spiritual and philosophical traditions, analysts can deepen their understanding of human suffering and renewal. They can create spaces in which questions of meaning, belonging, and grace are not pathologized but welcomed.

In these spaces, the analyst does not offer answers. They offer presence. They offer the possibility of a relationship in which suffering can be spoken, heard, and held without being resolved. They offer a place where the analysand can confront not only their symptoms but their existence – their longings, their fears, their search for a life worth living.

This is a practice that requires more than technical competence. It requires ethical and existential maturity. It requires the analyst to undergo their own process of becoming, to engage with their own suffering and questions, to cultivate the humility and patience necessary to accompany others on their journeys.

Dwelling with the Human: Psychoanalysis Beyond Technique

In a world increasingly driven by speed, efficiency, and distraction, psychoanalysis offers something precious: slowness, attention, care. It invites us to dwell with what is difficult, to remain present with what is painful, to honor the mystery and complexity of human life. This is not a luxury. It is an ethical necessity.

The future of psychoanalysis will belong to those who can hold this space – to those who refuse to trade presence for productivity, ambiguity for certainty, care for efficiency. It will belong to those who recognize that in listening deeply to another person's suffering, something sacred is preserved.

As we consider the trajectory of psychoanalysis in the decades to come, one essential truth emerges: the future of this practice will not be secured through institutional expansion, technological integration, or professional recognition alone. It will be secured through the quality of the encounter between analyst and analysand – through the capacity of analysts to remain steadfast in their commitment to human depth, ethical presence, and the irreducibility of suffering.

This is a future that demands more than theoretical sophistication. It demands analysts who are willing to risk their own comfort, to relinquish the illusion of mastery, to enter fully into the lived realities of those who come seeking help. It demands analysts who can tolerate the discomfort of ambiguity, who can remain present in the face of suffering without defense or distraction.

The cultivation of such analysts will require a reorientation of training and education. Rather than focusing solely on technical skill acquisition or theoretical memorization, analytic training must foreground the ethical, philosophical, and spiritual dimensions of the work. Candidates must be encouraged not only to learn but to become – to undergo their own analytic journeys, to confront their own histories, to grapple with the questions that animate human existence.

In this context, the integration of contemporary psychoanalysis will be vital. As the cultural fragmentation of meaning continues to accelerate, patients will increasingly bring into the analytic space not only their psychological wounds but also their existential longings. They will bring questions of belonging, grace, rupture, and renewal – questions that cannot be answered by clinical technique alone.

The analyst who is prepared to meet these questions will not do so with doctrine or dogma but with presence and humility. They will understand that healing does not reside in explanation but in encounter. They will recognize that the analytic space is one of the few remaining places where the human soul can be taken seriously – where suffering is neither pathologized nor dismissed but engaged with, with care and reverence.

This is a demanding future. It requires analysts who are willing to dwell in uncertainty, who are able to accompany others without imposing their own agendas, who are attuned to the ethical stakes of their work. But it is also a hopeful future. For in this work, something essential is preserved: the dignity of human suffering, the possibility of transformation, the affirmation of presence over product.

Psychoanalysis will not survive because it has adapted to the demands of the marketplace or the metrics of efficiency. It will survive because there remain those who believe in the value of deep listening, of ethical presence, of human care. It will survive because there remain those who are willing to do the slow, difficult, and essential work of being with others in their suffering.

And in that work, psychoanalysis will continue to bear witness to the enduring mystery of what it means to be human.

Állos is not just a word. It is the soul of the analytic vocation. It reminds us that to know another is not to possess them, and to be known is not to be exposed, but to be held. Psychoanalysis that forgets the sacredness of the other becomes technique. But psychoanalysis that remembers *állos* becomes liturgy – an embodied practice of reverent listening, of presence in the face of suffering, of remaining where no answers suffice.

In the end, to become a psychoanalyst in the key of *állos* is to give oneself to a kind of unknowing: to stand at the threshold between suffering and meaning, and to become, in the words of the Gospel, "another advocate."

Állos and the Alienist: Estrangement, Otherness, and the Origins of Healing

The word *állos* – "another of a different kind" – echoes not only through theology and philosophy, but through the very origins of modern clinical practice. The alienist, a term largely displaced today by "psychiatrist" or "psychotherapist," was once the primary designation for the physician of the mentally ill. The term emerged from the French *aliéniste*, derived from *aliéner*, meaning "to alienate" or "to estrange," and ultimately from the Latin *alienus* – foreign, other, belonging to another.

This lineage is no coincidence. To be *mentally ill* – in the pre-modern and early modern imagination – was to be othered. One was no longer at home in oneself, no longer "of sound mind," no longer belonging to the shared social world. The alienist, then, was not simply a physician of the brain, but a mediator between worlds: between reason and unreason, society and exclusion, sameness and otherness. At its roots, the alienist was the one who met the one who had become *állos* to themselves and to others.

Estrangement as Symptom and Signal

The early alienist operated in an ambiguous space: part custodian, part physician, part exile themselves. Philippe Pinel, often credited with liberating the 'mad' from their chains in 18th-century France, was both a humanitarian and an administrator of social order. He used the term *manie sans délire* (mania without delusion) to describe certain forms of moral madness – suggesting that even without loss of reason, one could become psychically *othered*, morally displaced.

What psychoanalysis inherits from this tradition is a double awareness: that alienation is not simply a symptom, but a structure of human experience. Freud himself spoke of the *uncanny* (*das Unheimliche*), that which is strangely familiar and disturbingly close. To suffer psychologically is not merely to feel pain – it is to feel estranged from one's own thoughts, body, past, or potential. The alienist – and later the psychoanalyst – encounters this estrangement not only as pathology but as ontological event.

Here we find the deep kinship between *állos* and the role of the analyst. The patient arrives not simply as one suffering from symptoms, but as one estranged from their speech, their desire, their capacity to love or grieve. And the analyst must not try to 'normalize' too quickly, for it is precisely in the zone of alienation where truth begins to emerge. The analyst, like the alienist before them, must become familiar with what is foreign. They must become *at home in the exile* – to use a Winnicottian phrase that echoes this ethos.

From Alienation to Alterity: Psychoanalysis as Threshold

The shift from alienist to psychoanalyst marks more than a linguistic transition. It signals a move from viewing the patient as simply *othered* (in the sense of exclusion), to *othered* in the deeper phenomenological sense – as unknowable, complex, mysterious. The analyst no longer only treats the alienation but enters into it. The analytic space becomes a sanctuary for estrangement – a liminal field where the person may begin to re-approach themselves through the presence of another.

This is *állos* in practice: the analyst as another of a different kind. Not friend, not family, not preacher, not judge. But not neutral either. The analyst is a relational third – someone who stands beside the patient in their unhoming, their wandering, their half-spoken grief. The analyst does not cure alienation by erasing difference, but by accompanying the patient into and through it.

This work bears spiritual resonance. In Christian theology, Christ is described as both fully God and fully human – *another of a different kind*, who enters the human condition not to erase its suffering, but to suffer with. The alienist, in its most ancient sense, becomes a proto-icon of the priest, the shepherd, the prophet who risks closeness to the one whom society has cast off.

Psychoanalysis at its best recovers this radical relationality. And theological psychoanalysis – in particular, the vision of Állos Theological Seminary – restores this sacred function. Not by returning to clerical authority, but by recognizing that to be with the other in their alienation is already a form of ministry.

Analyst as Alienist

To carry forward the legacy of the alienist is to adopt a posture of reverent strangeness. The contemporary psychoanalyst is not one who has mastered the psyche, but one who has been undone by it. They are not immune to alienation – they have known it. And in knowing it, they have learned how to stand beside it without fear. They become, in a real sense, *another advocate* (*állos paraklētos*) – the one who listens without rushing to solve, who dwells where others flee.

References

American Psychiatric Association. (2000). *Diagnostic and statistical manual of mental disorders* (4th ed., Text Revision). Washington, DC: Author.

American Psychiatric Association. (2013). *Diagnostic and statistical manual of mental disorders* (5th ed.). Arlington, VA: Author.

Aquinas, T. (1997). *Summa theologiae: A concise translation*. New York: Thomas More Publishing.

Beebe, J. (2005). *Integrity in depth*. College Station, TX: Texas A&M University Press.

Benjamin, J. (2007). *Intersubjectivity, thirdness, and mutual recognition*. https://icpla.edu/wp-content/uploads/2013/03/Benjamin-J.-2007-ICP-Presentation-Thirdness-present-send.pdf.

Bion, W. R. (1962). *Learning from experience*. London: Heinemann.

Bion, W.R. (1970). *Attention and interpretation*. London: Tavistock Publications.

Bion, W. R. (1992). *Cogitations*. London: Karnac Books.

Bion, W. R. (2019). *War memoirs 1917–1919*. London: Routledge.

Boss, M. (1977). *Existential foundations of medicine and psychology*. New York: Jason Aronson.

Brentano, F. (1995). *Psychology from an empirical standpoint*. London: Routledge.

Briefwechsel, 1918–1969. Marbach am Neckar, Germany: Schillergesellschaft.

Cady, H. E. (2014). *The spiritual writings of H. Emilie Cady*. Jazzybee Verlag.

Camus, A. (1989). *The stranger*. New York: Vintage Books.

Camus, A. (1991). *The fall*. New York: Vintage Books.

Camus, A. (1992). *The rebel: An essay on man in revolt*. New York: Vintage Books.

Camus, A. (2007). *Exile and the kingdom*. New York: Vintage Books.

Camus, A. (2018). *The myth of Sisyphus*. New York: Knopf Doubleday Publishing Group

Charles, M. (2017). *Introduction to contemporary psychoanalysis: Defining terms and building bridges*. London: Routledge.

Cieri, F. & Esposito, R. (2019). Psychoanalysis and neuroscience: The bridge between mind and brain. *Brain. Frontiers in Psychology*, 10(1790) https://www.ncbi.nlm.nih.gov/pmc/articles/PMC6724748/.

Civitarese, G. (2019). On Bion's concepts of negative capability and faith. *Psychoanalytic Quarterly*, 88:751–783.

Das, S. (1997). *Awakening the Buddha within*. New York: Broadway Books.

DeRobertis, E. (2008). *Humanizing child developmental theory: A holistic approach*. Bloomington, IN: iUniverse Inc.

Eigen, M. (1985). Toward Bion's starting point: Between catastrophe and faith. *International Journal of Psychoanalysis*, 66:321–330.

Eigen, M. (1986). *The psychotic core*. Northvale, NJ: Jason Aronson.

Eigen, M. (1992). *Coming through the whirlwind*. Wilmette, IL: Chiron.

Eigen, M. (1993). *The electrified tightrope*. Northvale, NJ: Jason Aronson.

Eigen, M. (1999). *Toxic nourishment*. London: Karnac Books.

Eigen, M. (2001). *Damaged bonds*. London: Karnac Books.

Eigen, M. (2005). *Emotional storm*. Littletown, CT: Wesleyan University Press.

Eigen, M. (2006). Faith and disillusionment: An interview with Dr. Michael Eigen. *Dharma Cafe*. http://www.dharmacafe.com/index.php/life-cycles/article/faith-and- disillusionment-an-interview-with-dr-michael-eigen/.

Eigen, M. (2011a). *Contact with the depths*. London: Karnac Books.

Eigen, M. (2011b, November). Beauty and destruction: Can goodness survive life, and what would that mean?First Humanities Forum. Lecture conducted from Busan, Korea.

Eigen, M. (2011). *Contact with the depths*. London: Karnac Books.

Eigen, M. (2012). *Kabbalah and psychoanalysis*. London: Routledge.

Eigen, M. (July 26, 2013). Personal communication.

Eigen, M. (2014). *Faith*. London: Routledge.

Eigen, M. (2021). *Eigen in Seoul*, volume 3: Pain and beauty, terror and wonder. London: Routledge.

Eigen, M. (2021). *Eigen in Seoul: Faith and transformation*. London, UK: Routledge.

Fink, A. (2000). The role of the researcher in the qualitative research process. A potential barrier to archiving qualitative data. *Forum Qualitative Sozialforschung*, 1(3). https://www.researchgate.net/publication/45346178_The_Role_of_the_Researcher_in_the_Qualitative_Research_Process_A_Potential_Barrier_to_Archiving_Qualitative_Data.

Frankl, V. (2006). *Man's search for meaning*. Boston, MA: Beacon Press.

Frankl, A. (2019). *The doctor and the soul: From psychotherapy to logotherapy*. New York: Vintage Books.

Frankl, V. (2021). *Yes to life: In spite of everything*. Boston, MA: Beacon Press.

Freud, S. (1909). *Family romances*. S.E., 9:235–244. London: Hogarth Press.

Freud, S. (1900). *Interpretation of dreams*, S.E., 4–5. London: Hogarth Press.

Freud, S. (1913). *Totem and taboo*, S.E., 13: 1–161. London: Hogarth Press.

Freud, S. & Breuer, J. (2004). *Studies in hysteria*. London: Penguin Classic. (Original work Published 1895).

Gadamer, H.-G. (2013). *Truth and method*. London: Bloomsbury Academic.

Ghosh, S. (2020). Perichoresis. *Alchetron*. https://alchetron.com/Perichoresis.

Grotstein, J. (2013). *Who is the dreamer who dreams the dream? A study of psychic presences*. London: Routledge.

Hanh, T. N. (2014). *No mud, no lotus: The art of transforming suffering*. Berkeley, CA: Parallax Press.

Heidegger, M. (1966). *Discourse on thinking*. New York: Harper & Row.

Heidegger, M. (1977). *The question concerning technology and other essays*. New York: Harper & Row Publishers.

Heidegger, M. (1978). Letter on humanism. In D. F. Krell (Ed.), *Basic Writings*. London: Routledge.

Heidegger, M., Blochmann, E., & Storch, J. (1989). *Martin Heidegger*, Elisabeth Blochmann:

Heidegger, M. (1996). *Being and time*. (J. Stambaugh, Trans.). New York: State University of New York Press. (Original work published 1927).

Heidegger, M. (2000). *Introduction to metaphysics*. New Haven, CT: Yale University Press.

Heidegger, M. (2002). *Identity and difference*. Chicago: University of Chicago Press.

Heidegger, M. (2003). *Philosophical and political writings*. New York: Continuum International Publishing Group, Ltd.

Heidegger, M. (2004). *Letters 1925–1975: Hannah Arendt and Martin Heidegger*. New York: Harcourt, Inc.

Hicks, S. R. C. (2004). *Explaining postmodernism: Skepticism and socialism from Rousseau to Foucault*. Scholargy Publishing.

Hillman, J. (1996). *The soul's code: In search of character and calling*. New York, NY: Random House.

Hillman, J. (1998). *Suicide and the soul*. Washington, DC: Spring Publications.

The Holy Bible, New International Version. (1984). Grand Rapids, MI: Zondervan Publishing House.

James, W. (2018). *The varieties of religious experience*. Chicago, IL: Anonymous Press. (Original work published 1902).

Jung, C. G. (1981). *The archetypes and the collective unconscious*. In R.F.C Hull (Ed. & Trans.), Collected works of C.G. Jung (Vol. 9, Part 1). Princeton, NJ: Princeton University Press. (Original work published 1968).

Jung, C. G. (2003). *Four archetypes*. London: Routledge.

Keiser, J. (2021). A brain researcher on what Freud got right. https://www.washingtonpost.com/entertainment/books/a-brain-researcher-on-what-freud-got-right/2021/02/25/42ed23a6-7544-11eb-948d-19472e683521_story.html.

Kierkegaard, S. (1983). *Sickness unto death*. In Hong, W & Hong, E (Ed & Trans). *Kierkegaard's Writings*, 19. Princeton, NJ: Princeton University Press. (Original work published 1846). (Original work published 1849).

Kierkegaard, S. (1986). *Fear and trembling*. New York: Penguin Books. (Original work published 1843).

Kierkegaard, S. (1992). Concluding unscientific postscript to philosophical fragments, Volume 1. In Hong, W & Hong, E (Ed & Trans) *Kierkegaard's Writings*, Vol 12.1. Princeton, NJ: Princeton University Press. (Original work published 1846).

Kierkegaard, S. (1992b). Concluding unscientific postscript to philosophical fragments, Volume 1. In Hong, W & Hong, E (Ed & Trans) *Kierkegaard's Writings*, Vol 12.1. Princeton, NJ: Princeton University Press. (Original work published 1846).

Kierkegaard, S. (2009). *Upbuilding discourses in various spirits.* In Hong, W & Hong, E (Ed &Trans) *Kierkegaard's Writings*, Vol 15. Princeton, NJ: Princeton University Press. (Original work published 1847).

Knafo, D. (2018). Beginnings and endings: Time and termination in psychoanalysis. *Psychoanalytic Psychology*, 1, 8–14. https://www.apa.org/pubs/journals/features/pap-pap0000125.pdf.

Laing, R. D. (1965). *The divided self.* London: Penguin Books.

Mate, G. (2011). *When the body says no: Exploring the stress-disease connection*. Indianapolis, IN: Wiley Publishing.

McGowan, K. (2014). The second coming of Sigmund Freud. https://www.discovermagazine.com/mind/the-second-coming-of-sigmund-freud.

McWilliams, N. (2011). *Psychoanalytic diagnosis: Understanding personality structure in the clinical process* (2nd ed.). New York: Guilford Press.

Mitchell, S. (1988). *Relational concepts in psychoanalysis: An integration.* Cambridge, MA: Harvard University Press.

The NAS New Testament Greek Lexicon. (n.d.). *Bible Study Tools.* Retrieved from http://www.biblestudytools.com/lexicons/greek/nas/aphiemi.html.

Nietzsche, F. (1974). *The gay science: With a prelude in rhymes and an appendix of songs.* New York: Vintage Books. (Original work published 1882).

Nietzsche, F. (1989). *On the genealogy of morals and ecce homo.* New York: Vintage Books. (Original work published 1888).

Nietzsche, F. (1990). *The twilight of the idols and the Anti-Christ: or how to philosophize with a hammer.* London: Penguin Classics. (Original work published in 1889).

Nietzsche, F. (1996). *Human, all too human: A book for free spirits.* Lincoln, NE: Bison Books. (Original work published 1878).

Nietzsche, F. (2022). *Thus spake Zarathustra: A book for all and none.* Honiton, UK: Notting Hill Editions. (Original work published 1883).

Novich, J. & Novich, K. (2006). *Good goodbyes: Knowing how to end in psychotherapy and Psychoanalysis.* New York: Jason Aronson.

Ogden, T. (1989). *The primitive edge of experience.* Lanham, MD: Rowman & Littlefield Publishers.

Ogden, T. (1992). *The primitive edge of experience.* Lanham, MD: Rowman & Littlefield Publishers, Inc.

Orange, D. (2014). And we shall be changed: To hold theory lightly is to surrender assumptions: Discussion of clinical narrative by Steven Stern. *International Journal of Psychoanalytic Self Psychology* 9(3). https://www.resea

rchgate.net/publication/264090536_And_We_Shall_Be_Changed_To_Hold_Theory_Lightly_Is_to_Surrender_Assumptions_Discussion_of_Clinical_Narrative_by_Steven_Stern.

Oxford Reference. (2021). Negative capability. https://www.oxfordreference.com/view/10.1093/oi/authority.20110803100227203.

Potter, B. (2017). Epilogue. In M. Dezelic (Ed.), *Trauma treatment – healing the whole person: Meaning-Centered Therapy and trauma treatment foundational phase-work manual.* Gables, FL: Presence Press International.

Potter, B. (2018). Tropisms of creative faith and destructiveness in the works of Michael Eigen and Martin Heidegger. In S. Block & L. Daws (Eds.), *Living moments: On the work of Michael Eigen* (pp. 65–81). New York: Routledge.

Potter, B. (2018a). *Elements of self-destruction.* London: Routledge.

Potter, B. (2018b) *Elements of reparation: Truth, faith, and transformation in the works of Heidegger, Bion, and Beyond.* London: Routledge.

Potter, B. (2023). *Faith sense and sensibility in the psychoanalytic treatment process: A phenomenological psychoanalytic study* [Unpublished doctoral dissertation]. Institute of Contemporary Psychoanalysis.

Schlesinger, H. (2016). *Endings and beginnings: On terminating psychotherapy and psychoanalysis.* London: Routledge.

Schneider, K. (2007). *Existential-integrative psychotherapy: Guideposts to the core of practice.* London: Routledge.

Shapira-Berman, O. (2021) At the beginning, there was… re-considering the concepts of 'faith' and 'trust' as analytic objects. *Contemporary Psychoanalysis* 57:506–536.

Solms, M. (2018). The neurobiological underpinnings of psychoanalytic theory and therapy. *Frontiers in Behavioral Neuroscience.* https://www.frontiersin.org/articles/10.3389/fnbeh.2018.00294/full.

Stenstad, G. (2006). *Transformations: Thinking after Heidegger*(New Studies Phenomenology / Hermeneutics). Madison, WI: University of Wisconsin Press.

Stolorow, R. & Atwood, G. (1996). The intersubjective perspective. *Psychoanalytic Review,* 83, 181–194. https://icpla.edu/wp-content/uploads/2012/10/Stolorow-Atwood-The-Intersubjective-Perspective-Psychoa.-Review-1996.pdf.

Symington, J & N. (1996). *The clinical thinking of Wilfred Bion.* London: Karnac Books.

Walter, A. (2017). How to be a servant leader in your family. https://www.viewfromthetop.com/blog/how-to-be-a-servant-leader-in-your-family.

Winnicott, D. W. (1988). *Human nature.* New York: Shocken Books.

Zirogiannis, M. (2018). *A quote a day.* Morrisville, NC: Lulu.com

Index

Made in the USA
Las Vegas, NV
19 September 2026

04716648-75d7-454b-bce6-bbdd1decb3baR01